HEALTH
AND
SOCIETY

JOHN P. DOLAN
and
WILLIAM N. ADAMS-SMITH

HEALTH AND SOCIETY

A Documentary History
of Medicine

A Continuum Book
THE SEABURY PRESS, NEW YORK

014530

1978
The Seabury Press
815 Second Avenue
New York, New York 10017

Printed in the United States of America

Library of Congress Cataloging in Publication Data
Dolan, John Patrick.   Health and society.
(A Continuum book)
Bibliography: p. 223
Includes index.
1. Medicine—History.   2. Medicine—History—Sources.
I. Adams-Smith, William N., 1929–   joint author.
II. Title. [DNLM: 1. History of medicine. WZ40 D659h]
R131.D64   610'.9   77–13478   ISBN 0–8164–9324–3

TO ALL WHO THROUGHOUT HISTORY HAVE DEDICATED
THEMSELVES TO THE PRESERVATION OF HEALTH
AND THE PREVENTION OF DISEASE

Contents

Preface

THE PRESENT VOLUME is an attempt to present the history of medicine in a concise manner that places it within the overall social and cultural context of the past. By combining the crafts of the teaching physician with those of the historian, we have sought to reach a balance in narrating the ever-changing flow of history and illuminating the unchanging aim of all medicine—the elimination of human suffering.

Unlike traditional accounts of the history of medicine, which often are little more than cumbersome catalogues of the great doctors and their achievements, the authors have incorporated into the text the basic writings of those who made major contributions to the art and science of healing. In this way, they hope to make their account come alive by allowing the great personalities to speak for themselves. The inclusion of documents is based upon the conviction that no one can comprehend the task of the physician without some knowledge of the sources of his profession.

In order to demonstrate the great variety of the sources of medicine, we have provided a wide range of authors, both thinkers and doers, philosophers and scientists. Because medicine is an integral part of social and cultural history, selections from literary figures as well as government documents and surveys also are included. The selected texts are lengthy enough to provide real substance for study and analysis.

The physician is well aware that he cannot treat a patient without a medical history; yet it is equally important that the practitioner have an adequate knowledge of the origins and development of his profession. The medical profession in Western civilization is of rather recent origin, whereas the study and practice of medicine can be traced to prehistoric times. Today, there is growing criticism about profitism in American medical practice. If the physician and the public were more aware of the great contribution of medicine to civilization, much of the acrimony of the critics and much of the defensiveness of the accused would be lessened. Here again, history plays an important role.

One of the major difficulties in understanding medicine today is the multiplicity of seemingly unrelated facts and details. Like the complexities of modern-day living itself, it often defies explanation. It is the task of history to unravel this web of seeming incoherence by placing the achievements and the failures of medicine in proper perspective. Modern medicine is deeply involved in the treatment of disease. Yet historically, its role was much wider—the elimination of all human suffering. Although medicine today is regarded as being largely scientific and empiric, it is nonetheless dependent for its functioning upon attitudes and philosophies that are deeply rooted in the past. For example, the current idea of disease as a special kind of entity that can be controlled and eventually eliminated may be but a passing product of the historical process. For many centuries, disease and sickness were regarded as afflictions of the gods, supernatural phenomena. Throughout most of Western history, it was firmly believed that health depended on four humors—blood, phlegm, black bile, and yellow bile; four temperaments—sanguine, phlegmatic, choleric, and melancholic; and their reaction to the environment. Yet today the notion of disease as an entity is being challenged. The image of disease as a thing has taken on a new identity, and is now widely regarded as being an altered bodily state or condition. Thus, in a certain sense, the ancient humoral theory of a balance between various forces has been curiously revitalized. This shift of meaning would be unintelligible without a knowledge of the constant revisionism of medical opinion reflected in its history.

The same observation is valid in pointing out that what today is called scientific medicine is in fact more properly called medical technology, often quite unscientific. The idea of science as it was understood in the nineteenth century simply does not apply anymore, nor does what it meant to the ancient Greeks and Romans.

To present five thousand years of medicine in a single volume demands a policy of strict selectivity. Many important names have been sacrificed in an effort to represent the major figures and movements. For this reason, we have included a listing of selected material for further reading for each chapter. The book also contains a chronology of great medical events throughout history.

HEALTH
AND
SOCIETY

1

Prehistory and Ancient Civilizations

THERE HAS ALWAYS been a great deal of speculation about the beginnings of medicine. Various writers have suggested that Paleolithic man would have responded to injury in an instinctive way, for example, immobilizing a fracture or putting a compress on a wound. A comparison has been made with animals that assist one of their kind when ill or injured. However, there is no real evidence of any Paleolithic medicine. It is not until the New Stone Age, which began in Europe seven to ten thousand years ago, that we find actual evidence of medical practice. There is also evidence to suggest that Neolithic man used the water of mineral springs in the treatment of disease. Archaeological excavations have exposed large wooden pipes from this period in the vicinity of highly mineralized streams that did not need to be used for drinking water, as there was an abundance in the immediate vicinity.

It is interesting to note that whenever man invented some method of writing down his traditions there is a highly developed methodology explaining the phenomena of nature, including disease. These explanations invariably have a religious or magical character and are so similar in all ancient civilizations that one can only assume that once man reached a certain stage, faced with the same natural phenomena, he came spontaneously to similar explanations of these phenomena.

Primitive tribes today have much the same traditions. They accept coughs, colds, fevers, and rheumatism as regular occurrences, and these are treated by the patient or by members of the family using domestic remedies. A distinction is made between these and serious ailments, which are mysterious and cannot be cured by simple reme-

1

dies. They are therefore given a magical or religious significance. Such sickness required the intervention of a priest or a medicine man. One must stress that in the primitive mind there are no sharp differences among magic, religion, and medicine.

In the prevention of disease, primitive people very often reacted in a very common-sense manner, but to be accepted by the bulk of the population, this had to be disguised with magical or religious significance. For example, not only dead people but their clothing and othe possessions were considered dangerous, and the same was true of many sick people. Most primitive peoples would leave a region where a contagious disease had broken out, and although this might help in protection, more protection might be achieved by having nothing at all to do with the sick or dead. In many cases, the person who died, the hut in which he lived, and all his possessions were burned.

Among primitive peoples, two basic attitudes can be observed toward the crippled, aged, and sick. Some treat them kindly, feed them, attend to them, honor the aged, and make the necessary payments to have the sick person treated. Others, however, either abandon their handicapped members or kill them and sometimes eat them. It would be easy to assume that the latter type of behavior was found among more primitive societies, but this, in fact, was not the case. Food-gathering and fishing-and-hunting communities tend to treat their handicapped members well; whereas in societies where social organizations and property relations were more complex, the infirm were treated with much less sympathy. This oversimplification allows us to draw an interesting parallel with respect for life that is found in pastoral and urban communities today. In some societies, it was the custom for the infirm to ask to be killed. This was an early form of euthanasia carried out from respect and compassion for the sick person.

Before we condemn the primitive medicine man too vigorously, we should remember that because the cause of the disease was believed to be either magical or religious any effective treatment would have to have a considerable element of magic or religion in it. Because of the beliefs of the society in which he lived, the primitive medicine man considered it perfectly logical to employ magic or religion in reaching a diagnosis and in undertaking treatment. However, the magical or religious treatments were usually combined with some form of treatment that we would consider rational, such as poulticing, bloodletting, massage, vapor baths, or counterirritation. All of these treatments have been widely found among primitive societies. The evidence from extant, primitive societies indicates that the vast majority of medicine men were very sincere in their practices.

EGYPTIAN MEDICINE

The ancient Egyptians recognized three types of healers: the physician, the priest of Sekhmet (the goddess of Pestilence), and the sorcerer. Priests other than those of Sekhmet could be involved. Religion was concerned with the worship of gods or of the dead, and major illnesses were considered to be afflictions resulting from some offense committed against a god or an ancestor. Prevention and cure consisted of wearing amulets, reciting incantations, and performing certain rites. Texts of incantations and descriptions of other magic procedures are to be found in a variety of papyri. There were specific incantations for all aspects of health—for example, the protection of infants or the facilitation of childbirth—or against specific diseases.

Existing with magical and religious medicine was a strong practice of empirical and rational medicine, which does not appear to have grown from religious or magical medicine but rather to have developed concurrently during the Pyramid Age. There are some very important papyri that present the rational medical and surgical treatments of a variety of conditions and that indicate that physicians in Egypt practiced medicine of a far higher standard than is commonly realized.

The earliest medical literature of Egypt consisted of monographs, each of which was devoted to one particular subject. Later, such monographs were frequently combined to form compendiums. The three oldest known papyri are examples of such monographs. Unfortunately, there is nothing but small fragments of the first two, which were written about 1900 B.C. The papyrus of Kahun shows us that there was veterinary medicine in ancient Egypt and also that veterinary medicine had the same character as human medicine. The monograph deals with the diseases of various animals, for example: "Treatment for a bull with wind." The text follows a pattern that is found in other medical papyri. It begins with a title indicating the disease, which is named after its chief symptom. Then the other symptoms are indicated and prescriptions are given in some detail.

Most of the treatment is fully rational. For example, in one instance, the animal is sprinkled with cold water, rubbed with the juices of gourds or melons, fumigated, and, most important of all, venesection is performed on the nose and the tail, interestingly the two favorite places for venesection on cattle today. The disease described in this monograph is believed to be malign catarrhal fever, a cattle disease that has a high mortality.

The gynecological papyrus of Kahun is also a fragment from a monograph. There are three pages, the first two devoted to the presentation of seventeen cases, each of which follows the same pattern: "Remedy for a woman who suffers from . . ." followed by a list of symptoms.

The next section, pathogenetic rather than diagnostic, is introduced by the formula "Thou shalt say concerning it . . ." and here the cause of the symptom is indicated—the uterus has gone up or down, is biting or starving and restless.

And finally the treatment is indicated, beginning with the words "Thou shalt do against it. . . ." The third page of the papyrus is devoted to prescriptions concerned with pregnancy. There are prescriptions intended to enable one to find out whether a woman is fertile or barren, whether she has conceived, what the sex of the fetus is, and for promoting or preventing conception.

The Edwin Smith papyrus is a monograph on wounds and is therefore a surgical text. The Ebers papyrus is a collection of medical books dealing primarily with internal diseases. For the most part, it is a collection of recipes. Both papyri were written about 1600 B.C., but both are copies of much older texts that go back to the Pyramid Age. The Smith papyrus contains fragments from an earlier book on the vessels of the heart; some incantations against pests; and a prescription for women's diseases, cosmetic recipes, and an ailment of the anus, but the bulk of the papyrus is concerned with wounds. It describes forty-eight cases: injuries, fractures, wounds, dislocations, tumors. This monograph is arranged systematically, the cases being listed in order from the head to the feet. In the Smith papyrus, we find an elaboration of the pattern that we first came across in the gynecological papyrus of Kahun. The title is usually brief and named after the chief symptom, then detailed instructions to the surgeon, advising him in examining the case, palpating the wound, probing it. It tells him what symptoms he should look for, listing, describing, and evaluating them in a way not encountered in any other archaic medical book. The examination is followed by the diagnosis, which as a rule is the repetition of the title followed by the verdict.

Although, strictly speaking, the verdict is not a prognosis, it implicitly includes one, and if the verdict is that the ailment is not to be treated, we encounter the viewpoint, widespread in antiquity, that hopeless cases were not to be touched. After the verdict comes the treatment. Any manipulations that are required are usually described as part of the examination, and the treatment that follows the verdict consists mainly of the application of dressings, occasionally the use of the cautery, and indicates the general nursing and dietetic measures to be employed. In some cases, several diagnoses are given. There may be as many as five different findings following the examination of a particular wound, and the verdict and treatment vary according to the findings. Careful consideration is given to the various possibilities that the course of a particular wound may take.

Although the Ebers and the Edwin Smith papyri date from the first half of the sixteenth century B.C. and were probably found in the same tomb, they differ in many ways. The Ebers papyrus is a great deal longer and is a complete compendium of medicine with a clearly defined beginning. Moreover, the Edwin Smith papyrus is devoted to a monograph on wounds, while the Ebers papyrus is a collection of monographs and excerpts on a variety of subjects. It has three main parts, the first of which is on medicine and surgery, but the type of minor surgery that could only have been dealt with by a general practitioner. The surgical section deals with enlarged lymphatic glands, abscesses, and swellings. The medical section is a book on "Diseases of the Cardia," containing descriptions of disease syndromes with instructions for their treatment. This collection follows the same pattern as the Smith papyrus. The second group of texts is a textbook of physiology. It comprises two extremely important theoretical treatises on the heart and the vessels. The third and largest group of texts consists of collections of recipes with prescriptions for the treatment of internal diseases; diseases of the eyes, the skin, and women; and other ailments. The recipes appear to have been jotted down in the order in which the physician learned them. Treatment by incantation is recommended in only twelve cases, most of which are regarded as hopeless.

The Hearst and Berlin papyri contain a variety of remedies, many of which are duplicated in the Ebers papyrus, and not a great deal of new material is introduced. One other papyrus of interest is the fragment of a monograph on "Remedies for the Diseases of the Anus." It is obviously a copy of a much older work. This monograph is of interest because it is known that there was one medical specialist who was given the colorful title of "guardian of the anus." It contains forty-one prescriptions with one incidental description of a disease followed by diagnosis and a favorable verdict.

It is also known that Egyptian physicians took a careful case history, first listening to what the patient said and then asking questions. This was followed by a careful inspection, and in the Smith and Ebers papyri, there are references to a pale or ruddy complexion, bloodshot eyes, burning or watery eyes, a contracted jaw, an open mouth, an erect phallus, or abnormal smells. The physician also inspected urine, feces, "what is lifted by cough," or blood. Palpation was considered important. Physicians noted the temperature of the skin and were quite skillful in assessing the pulse, which they considered an important aid in diagnosis. They also made extensive use of functional tests.

There is no doubt that drugs were the chief therapeutic agents in Egyptian empirico-rational medicine because the country was famous for its drugs and poisons. They were administered as potions, candy, little cakes, pills, or suppositories. There was not a liquid from oil to milk to beer that was not absorbed rectally. Enemas were employed regularly, usually in quantities of from one to three pints and containing all types of mild drugs. Inhalations were often used, and both anus and vagina were frequently fumigated. We do know that the properties of senna, castor oil, and opium were known to the Egyptians. A small number of minerals were used for ingestion or topical application. Surgeons reduced dislocations and aligned fractures and then splinted them or put them in a cast. Wounds were treated with applications of fresh meat that not only acted to stop hemorrhage by means of pressure but also contained hemostatic components. Cauterization was employed regularly and often poultices were applied. It is quite possible that wounds were sutured because infibulation was commonly practiced on young girls. Superficial tumors and cysts were removed, and abscesses were incised and drained.

It is of particular importance that we find, in the oldest medical literature dating to almost 3000 B.C., two theoretical treatises, one of which deals primarily with pathology and the other with physiology. The basic idea of both was that in the human body there was a system of vessels originating in the heart; connecting it with all the other parts of the body; and carrying air, liquids, such as blood, urine, tears, and sperm, and solid matter, such as feces, all believed to come from the heart. The heart was considered the central organ, and its beat was felt in the pulse; it was also the seat of thinking, feeling, and all nervous functions.

From the beginning of a united Egypt, there existed alongside the magical and religious rites for the sick a highly intellectual and systematic approach to empirical and rational medicine. We must give the Egyptians credit for treating medicine as a science as well as an art. Egyptian doctors were called to all the courts of the ancient world, and Egyptian medicine had a powerful influence, for example, in Persia and Greece, long after the decline of the Egyptian empire.

MESOPOTAMIAN MEDICINE

The history of Mesopotamia is much more complicated than that of Egypt because many peoples were involved; moreover although the country had natural boundaries, these were not so formidable as those of Egypt, and the country was much more open and vulnerable to nomads and marauders. Not only did Mesopotamia strongly influence its immediate neighbors, Palestine, Syria, Asia Minor, and Persia, but there also were early contacts with India and possibly even China. Waterborne diseases were common and so were various forms of dysentery. Typhoid fever is still frequent today, malaria was more common than in Egypt, and leprosy had occurred for generations. The custom of segregating lepers, so familiar to us from biblical references in Leviticus, originated in Mesopotamia. Extant medical texts make it evident that diseases of the respiratory tract, particularly acute and chronic bronchitis and pneumonia, were frequent. Moreover, Mesopotamia was on the highway between East and West and must have been prone to acute epidemic diseases.

Whereas in Egyptian medicine we could see the existence of empirico-rational medicine alongside magico-religious medicine, Mesopotamian medicine remained religious. Although the physicians of Mesopotamia, who in all cases were also priests, did use some empirical formulas, these were probably of Egyptian origin. Like the Egyptians, the Mesopotamians were very acute observers of physical signs, but all aspects of prognosis and treatment were heavily overlaid with religious and magical formulas. Although medicine was never able to free itself from religion, the law was divorced from religion. Gradually, the administration of the law was taken away from the priests entirely and placed in the hands of civil judges and secular courts. The code of Hammurabi was largely the law of torts and was particularly concerned with compensation for injury or damage. There is specific reference in the code to the reward given to, or retribution exacted from, surgeons. For the successful treatment of a serious wound or for a successful operation on the eye, the fee was ten shekels of silver if the patient was a patrician and five if he was a plebeian; for a slave, the owner paid two shekels. For the successful treatment of a broken bone or for the successful (surgical) treatment of an internal organ, the fee was five, three, or two shekels, respectively. If, however, an operation ended fatally or if an eye operation resulted in the loss of an eye, the physician's hands were cut off. We know from other civilizations that laws frequently remained on paper and were not applicable. They were formulated as a matter of policy and as a warning against abuse but if applied would have defeated their own purpose. Nevertheless, these laws are extremely interesting because they represent society's first attempt to protect itself against misuse of the physician's power, a power granted to him by society. The physician's liability for his actions was in every respect very similar to that of any other professional person entering into a contractual obligation.

HEBREW MEDICINE

Medicine among the Hebrews in biblical times and, to a greater degree, in the era of the Talmud was different from other early medical practices in other cultures. Although there are many references to physicians and medical practices in the Bible, such as Exodus 21:19, 2 Kings 8:29, 2 Chron. 16:12, and Jer. 8:22, none of these connects medicine exclusively with priesthood. Medicine was connected with religion only as far as it concerned public health matters. Public hygiene and individual prevention of disease were stressed.

Leviticus does not give the priests a monopoly on the practice of medicine but instead sets them up as guardians of public health against contagious diseases. The Essenes Asu who flourished from 200 B.C. until A.D. 100 united the knowledge of the priestly groups with popular medicine.

There is no written evidence of early medical literature because during those times all knowledge was transmitted orally. It is traditionally held that Enoch passed down all knowledge of the medicinal value of roots and herbs to Shem and Ebher. Another tradition is that Abraham passed his oral tradition to Moses, who in turn passed it to the prophets and King Solomon, who had it written down. The text was supposedly extant until the time of Hiskiya. The earliest Hebrew medical text that we have today is that of Assaf the Physician from the seventh century A.D. The contents are mainly derived from Greek and Oriental knowledge, but the Hebrew terms for disease and medicine and the ethics are of interest. There are no written records for early Hebrew medicine because writing was held in very high esteem, and once something was written down, it was considered sacred and unchangeable. Even in the ancient medical schools, all the studies were conducted orally.

Therefore, to piece together a picture of early Hebrew medicine, it is necessary to turn to Talmudic literature and other ancient literary sources.

The Bible mentions such diseases as fever, tuberculosis, jaundice, paralysis, and convulsions in 2 Kings 13:4; skin diseases in Lev. 13:14; internal diseases in Lev. 26:16; mental diseases in Deut. 28:28; and fevers in Deut. 28:22. From such evidence as this, the early medical practices can be more clearly understood.

The methods of treatment mentioned in the Bible are based on a clear understanding of nature. The medicines consisted of simple remedies rather than magical formulas as in other countries. Both the Bible and the Talmud contain many references warning against the use of magic in seeking cures. It would seem that the materia medica were obtained mainly from vegetables rather than from animals or minerals. There is a passage in Ben Sirach that states that "God makes remedies to grow out of the earth, and the wise man does not disdain them," which seems to give further credence to this practice.

Hebrew medical practices underwent a change after coming in contact with Babylonia, which stressed the use of incantations and magic. Such practices were adopted to a certain extent by the Hebrews as is shown both in the Bible in Dan. I and in the Talmud in Yer. Rosh Hash. I, 56d. Tobias and the Essenes cured through the use of prayers and incantations and were very influential in popular medicine. Another foreign influence on Hebrew medicine was Greek custom. There was a very large Jewish colony in Alexandria that was clearly open to Hellenistic influences, but the Jews never accepted the principles of Greek medicine.

The Jews were the first to formulate precepts concerning public and individual hygiene, which they closely related to ethical purity. The main categories of these precepts are the laws dealing with the Sabbath, the sabbatical year, the upkeep of the soil, ritual slaughter, isolation of people suffering from contagious diseases, the upkeep of shelter and garments, sexual practices and the purity of the race, work, and food. The Hebrews developed very advanced theories on infection and its transmission through animals, tableware, or anything with which the sick person would have been in contact. Practical medicine was taken away from the priests and also from any contact with magic to the extent that the punishment for practicing magic was death. However, it was in the area of pathological anatomy that the Hebrews were most advanced. Most of this was obtained from the practice of ritual slaughter and the requirements for ritually pure food. Jewish knowledge of anatomy was gathered from practical experience. If a slaughtered animal was found to be diseased, it was necessary to determine if the disease were serious enough to have caused the death of the animal within a year, in which case it would have been unfit for consumption. References to the fact that diseases were diagnosed from the condition of the organs appear several times in the Talmud, especially in the Tractate Hullin. These diagnoses were extremely clever and accurate in their perceptions because they were drawn from practical experience.

Jewish medicine was also highly advanced in the field of normal anatomy. Osteology was definitely more advanced in the Hebrew culture than it was in other cultures. Dissection of the human body was carried out by the pupils of Rabbi Ishmael, according to Bekh 45 and Nazir 52, referring to Thodos a physician. Special terms were developed to refer to the various diseases.

There was a great appreciation of the physician in Jewish society. He was respected as a messenger sent by God to help his fellowmen and had a much higher position than his counterparts in other cultures. In the Jerusalem Talmud, it is stated: "Honor thy physician even while thou needest him not" (Yer. Taan. 3). The physician played a respected role in the law courts, and permission had to be obtained to practice medicine. The physician also was held morally and financially responsible for his actions.

CHINESE MEDICINE

Chinese medicine has its origins in legend. The first legendary figures are Fu Hsi, to whom is attributed the *I Ching;* Shen Nung, the father of agriculture and herbal therapy; and Huang Ti, the creator of both ritual and medicine. The earliest medical text is the *Tao-chuan,* which dates from around 540 B.C. The first known doctor who was entirely separate from the priests and magicians was Pien Ts'io, who was thought to have lived from 430 B.C. to 350 B.C. He was already aware of the pulse rate and its importance in diagnosis and prognosis. The authorship of the *Nan Ching* has been attributed to him.

From 206 B.C. to A.D. 580, direct and/or indirect contact with Iran, India, Southeast Asia, and the Mediterranean was developed with the establishment of the Silk Road (122 B.C.) and the Burma Road (115 B.C.). Advances in medicine are reflected in the works of the Han empire, the *Nei-ching*—a classic of medicine; *Chin-fang*—collection of prescriptions; *Fang-chung*—sex and hygiene; and *Shan-sien*—methods and prescriptions for immortality. The *Nei-ching* is a classic treatise on internal medicine and supposedly the oldest medical book extant. In its present form, it dates from the eleventh century A.D. and is still considered a great authority. It contains many basic elements of Chinese medicine, the most important of which is the concept of yin and yang.

The Chinese belief in a dual power arose from attempts to explain creation, in which the final stage was the division of substance into a lighter part that rose to form heaven and a heavier part that sank to produce the earth. The two components of the dual power that arose from the primary state were called yin and yang. The original meaning of the two were cloudy and sunny, and their original function was the creation of heaven and earth; most of the connotations that they have gained can be logically derived from these original concepts.

Although yin represents the negative side and yang the positive, it must be remembered that both were always present. Neither exists in an absolute state, and one is always contained within the other. This interchange between yin and yang and the concept of duality contained within a single thing play important roles in Chinese medicine, and many examples can be found throughout the *Nei-ching*. According to the system proposed by the *Nei-ching*, man is divided into a lower region, a middle region, and an upper region, each of which is composed of one part yin and one part yang. Treatment of a specific disease or a specific organ depends on its location within a particular part of yin or yang. In regard to the human body, yang corresponds to the surface and yin the interior, and because both exist within the body, there is a similar relationship between the two in regard to the organs. A diagram of the relationship between the subdivisions of yin and yang and the various organs can be devised:

YANG	YIN
THE GREAT YANG	THE GREAT YIN
THE LESSER YANG	THE LESSER YIN
THE "SUNLIGHT"	THE ABSOLUTE YIN

the absolute yin includes the liver, the lesser yang includes the gall-bladder; the lesser yin includes the heart, the great yang includes the small intestines; the great yin includes the spleen, the sunlight includes the stomach; the great yin includes the lungs, the sunlight includes the lower intestines; the lesser yin includes the kidneys, the sunlight includes the bladder.

The affinity between yin and yang has a decisive role in man's health. Perfect harmony between the two means perfect health; disharmony leads to disease or death. This belief is exemplified in a chapter entitled: "Treatise on the Five Viscera in Relation to Their Part in Perfecting Life," which reads as follows:

The Heart is in accord with the pulse. The complexion of a person shows when the heart is in excellent condition. The heart rules over the kidneys.
The lungs are connected with the skin. The condition of the body hair shows when the lungs are in a good condition. The lungs rule over the heart.
The liver is connected with the muscles. The state of health of the liver

is determined by the condition of the finger and toe nails. The liver rules over the lungs.

The spleen is connected with the flesh. The lips indicate the condition of the stomach in their color and appearance. The liver rules over the lungs.

The kidneys are connected with the bones. The condition of the kidneys can be determined by the condition of the hair on the head. The kidneys rule over the spleen.

Hence if too much salt is used in food, the pulse hardens, tears appear, and the complexion changes. If too much bitter flavor is used in food, the skin becomes withered and the body hair falls out. If too much pungent flavor is used, the flesh hardens and wrinkles and the lips become slack. If too much sweet flavor is used, the bones ache and the hair on the head falls out. These then are the injuries which can be brought on by the five flavors.

We know that the heart craves the bitter flavor; the lungs crave the pungent flavor; the liver craves the sour flavor; the spleen craves the sweet flavor; and the kidneys crave the salty flavor. These are the proper combinations of the five flavors, and the state of the viscera can be observed by the appearance and color of their corresponding external organs.

When their color is green like grass they are without life; when it is yellow like that of lemons they are without life; when their color is black like coal they are without life; when their color is red like blood they are without life; when their color is white like old bones they are without life. This is how the five colors indicate death.

When the viscera are green like the kingfisher's wings they are filled with life; when they are red like a cock's comb they are filled with life; when they are yellow like the belly of a crab they are filled with life; when they are white like the grease of pigs they are full of life; and when they are black like the wings of a crow they are full of life. This is how the five colors manifest life.

The color of life displayed by the heart is like the red lining of a white silk robe; the color of life for the lungs is like the lucky red lining of a white silk robe; for the liver it is like the violet lining of a white silk robe; the color for the stomach is like the juniper berry colored lining; for the kidneys it is like the purple lining. These are the gorgeous external signs of life of the five viscera.

Each color and flavor belongs to one of the five viscera: white and the pungent flavor to the lungs; red and the bitter flavor to the heart; green and the sour flavor to the liver; yellow and the sweet flavor to the stomach; black and the salty flavor to the kidneys.

Thus white also belongs to the skin; red to the pulse; green to the muscles; yellow to the flesh; and black to the bones.

The pulse is connected with the eyes; the marrow with the brain; the muscles with the joints; the blood with the heart; the breath with the lungs.

The four limbs and their eight flexible joints are used from early morning until late at night. When people lie down to rest the blood returns to the liver. When the liver receives the blood it strengthens the vision. When the feet receive blood it strengthens the footsteps. When the palm receives the blood the hand is able to grasp. When the fingers receive the blood they are able to carry.

When a person is exposed to the wind, either while resting or walking, his blood will be affected. The blood then coagulates in the flesh and produces numbness in the hands and feet; when it coagulates within the pulse the blood ceases to flow; when it coagulates within the feet it produces pains and chills.

When the blood goes into these three organs and cannot return, its passage becomes empty and numbness and uncomfortableness result.

Man has twelve groups of large ducts and three hundred and sixty-four small ducts and twelve vessels of minor importance. They all protect the life-giving element and prevent evil influences from entering. When acupuncture is used it causes evil influences to leave.

At the beginning of an examination for disease one must find out whether the pulses of the five viscera are interrupted and one must control them. In order to know when to begin one must first establish which of the ten stems is to be the first month of the year.

The five indications that the functions of the five viscera are interrupted are the five pulses. Headaches and madness are indicated by an empty and sluggish lower pulse and a quick, full upper pulse. When diseases are examined at the pulse of the foot, it is felt they are in the region of the lesser Yin and the Great Yang, which indicates that they have also entered the kidneys.

Lack of discernment causes evil. Obscured eyesight and impaired hearing are indicated by a full lower pulse and an empty upper pulse. When these diseases are examined at the pulse of the foot, it is felt that they are in the region of the lesser Yang and the Great Yang; this indicates that the disease has entered the liver.

When the stomach is too full, dropsical swellings of the limbs, the diaphragm, the ribs and the flanks occur; then the pulse is disturbed below and flourishing above. If these diseases are examined at the pulse of the foot, one feels that they are in the region of the Sunlight and the Great Yang.

When there are pains at the heart and headaches the disease is located within the thorax. When these diseases are examined at the pulse of the hands, one feels that they are in the region of the Great Yang and the lesser Yin.

Thus it can be distinguished whether the pulses are large or small, slippery or rough, light or heavy. The external appearances of the five viscera can be put in the same categories.

The five viscera are connected with the five musical notes. The five colors can be used for subtle examinations and aid the eyes in the examination of diseases, and if one has the ability of combining the significance of the pulses with the significance of the colors a complete diagnosis can be made.

When the pulse has a red appearance and there is a persistent cough, the examiner says that there is amassed air in the heart and it is dangerous to eat. The disease is known as numbness of the heart. It is contracted through evil outside influences, causing anxiety and emptying the heart while the evil influences follow into it.

When the pulse has a white appearance and there is a light cough, the examiner can suspect that there is a mass of air in the thorax, causing shortness of breath and a hollow sound. The name of the disease is numbness of the lungs and the external signs are chills and fevers. This disease is caused by toxicity influencing the inner body.

When the pulse has a green appearance and the pulses at the left and right hands are pressed down for a long time, air is amassed within the heart and descends into the limbs and flanks. The disease is called numbness of the liver. It is contracted through chills and dampness and is associated with ruptures affecting the loins; then the feet hurt and the head aches.

When the pulse has a yellow appearance, the pulse becomes large and slow and air is massed in the spleen. The examiner will find that there is annoying gas. The disease is called rupture caused by troublesome gas. Women are also subject to this disease which can be contracted through exposure of perspiration on the four limbs to the wind.

When the pulse has a black appearance and the upper pulse is strong and big, the examiner will find that air is amassed in the small intestines, which is the region of Yin. The name of the disease is numbness of the kidneys. This illness can be cured by bathing in pure water and lying down to rest.

Every disease has a symbol through the variety of the five colors of the pulse. When the surface is yellow and the eyes see green, when the surface is yellow and the eyes see red, when the surface is yellow and the eyes see white, when the surface is yellow and the eyes see black, death will not come. But when the surface is green and the eyes see red, when the surface is red and the eyes see white, when the surface is green and the eyes see black, when the surface is black and the eyes see white, and when the surface is red and the eyes see green, death will come.

The period of Taoism, from the third century B.C. to the seventh century A.D., was dominated by the work of Ko Hung, a great alchemist and pathologist. His major works are the *Pao-p'u Tzu nei-wai-p'ien,* a treatise on alchemy, dietetics, and magic; *Chin-kuei-yo-fang,* the *Medications of the Golden Box;* and *Chou-hou pei-tai fang,* a collection of first-aid measures. Ko Hung developed a very clear idea of preventive medicine and formulated two rules for longevity—Tao Yin, a respiratory technique, and Fu-she, consumption of foods and drugs to augment the blood. He also recognized and described several diseases. In therapeutics, Ko Hung described many different and inexpensive drugs, developed the use of mineral materia medica, and encouraged research into immortality pills.

Another important figure of this period was Tao Hung-ching (452–536), who compiled the *Pen Ching*, a work dealing with three hundred and sixty-five mineral, herbal, and animal drugs.

In 624, the T'ai-i-shu, or Grand Medical Service, was organized to teach medicine under state supervision. Important works were written dealing with many diseases, ophthalmology, obstetrics, surgery, acupuncture, pediatrics, and materia medica. One of the outstanding monk-doctors of this age was Sun Szu-miao (581–682), author of *The Thousand Costly Recipes* and its supplement, *Treatise on Happiness, Articles on Hygiene, In the Depth of the Pillow, Exhaustive Study of the Silver Sea,* and *Treatise on Three Religions*. His medical system is a compromise between the Indian system of four elements and the Chinese doctrine of five viscera.

The most famous works of this age were compilations by Wang Ping. Other great classicists include Ch'ien Yi (1023–1104), the greatest pediatrician of his time; Sung Tz'u (1186–1249), the introducer of forensic medicine; and Wang Wei-i, composer of a compendium on acupuncture and creator of the men of bronze used as models for acupuncture. The Imperial College of Medicine was established in 1305, and medical encyclopedias were published. Four men were leaders in internal medicine: Liou Wan-su (1120–1200), Chang Tzu-ho (1156–1260), Li Tung-yuan (1179–1251), and Chou Tan-chi (1281–1358).

Medicine in other Asiatic countries was greatly influenced by Chinese medicine. Korea, Japan, and Vietnam share a common source of medical practice. The basic doctrines of these countries take a Chinese form, but they are not the same as classical Chinese. Korean medicine personalized Chinese medicine and added Indian data to it. Japan came in contact with Chinese medicine as early as 561 and continued the exchange for centuries. In Vietnam, Chinese medicine was taken and adapted to its different climate and available plants and animals.

The medicine of Central Asia has its own unique character. There are two separate aspects of Tibetan-Mongolian medicine—popular and scientific. Shamanism plays a major role in the popular medical practices, including the use of talismans, magical healing rites, and spells. Scientific medicine was centered in monasteries and religious schools that served as centers for learning and were equipped with libraries, dispensaries, and other learning aids. The books used for instruction were manuals translated from Sanskrit, Pali, Chinese, and traditional Tibetan works. The oldest of these books was the *Rgyud-bzi,* a basic work compiled in the eighth century. Tibetan medicine has a unique character because of the thermal springs, the abundant supply of materia medica, and its techniques. This is not to say that there are no foreign influences upon Tibetan medicine, but it retains a more individualistic character than the medicine of the other Asiatic countries.

MEDICINE IN ANCIENT PERSIA

As a general rule, physicians in ancient times did not need a license to practice. Anybody could claim to be an expert in matters of health and disease and treat sick people for a fee. This was modified by the Babylonians in that they protected society against malpractice of the surgeon by making him liable for his actions. In ancient Persia, however, there seems to have been some kind of licensing of surgeons. A Persian document dealing with the admission of physicians to the practice of surgery is the earliest preserved regulation of its kind.

Physicians practiced mostly as itinerants, just as the Greek doctors did at that time. The available evidence suggests that ancient Persian medicine was a blend of religious, magical, and empirical medicine. Incantations were widely used, although there was a good knowledge of the use of drugs. The armies of Persia needed surgeons, and there is no doubt that they knew how to treat battle wounds, perhaps just as well as their Greek and Babylonian colleagues because such techniques are easily learned from neighboring countries. All in all, it can be said that ancient Persia did not in any way contribute to the advancement of medicine. It did produce great rulers, great soldiers, and above all Zoroaster, a prophet and poet who taught a pure and highly ethical religion. Persia made its contribution to medicine much later, in the tenth and eleventh centuries A.D.

INDIAN MEDICINE

The Indo-Europeans had their period of archaic medicine, similar to that of the ancient Near East and consisting of empirical, religious, and magical elements. The separation of these three elements, which did not take place in Mesopotamia and was only begun in Egypt, became almost complete with Indo-Europe, particularly in Greece.

In both Greece and India, medicine became much more effective than it had ever been in Egypt and Mesopotamia because the Greeks and Indians acquired a much more profound knowledge of nature and of man within his environment. Both had forms of religious and magical medicine, but on the basis of empiricism, they developed philosophical systems of medicine that looked beyond the individual for laws of universal application.

Although there are striking similarities in the development of Greek and Indian medicine, there also are great differences. The Greek emphasized reason and logic; India also developed rational systems of medicine but included a mystic approach. The Greek approach paved the way for modern Western science, but Indian medicine was better prepared to handle mental and spiritual troubles, and its systems of meditation, particularly Yoga, provided therapeutic methods unknown to the West in antiquity.

Malaria was probably the chief health problem to India, not only because it kills and disables large numbers of people, but also because it saps vitality. It has been endemic in all parts of the country except the mountainous regions of Kashmir, Nepal, and Bhutan. The enteric diseases, such as dysentery and diarrhea, have been even more prevalent. Plague spread from rats to man, and cholera has been a major epidemic disease of India. It is highly probable that tuberculosis existed in ancient India as it did in the Mediterranean world. Leprosy must have been endemic in India from the earliest times. Like all tropical countries, India had a high incidence of worm diseases. Thus, we can see that India presented many and more serious health problems than Greece.

Because we have no literary records, our knowledge of the Indus civilization, like that of Crete, is derived entirely from archaeological findings. They are so rich, however, that they give us a picture of life in ancient India and also illustrate some aspects of great medical interest. We surmise that their medicine must have been similar to that of other people who were civilized in the third millennium B.C.—that is, a combination of religious, magical, and empirical rites and procedures. Amulets protected against evil, hence against disease; prayers were said to placate the gods; incantations were probably performed to drive out evil spirits; and, like all peoples, the inhabitants of the Indus Valley must have known drugs and household remedies with which to treat the sick. Almost all houses had bathrooms, which, although not uncommon in Egypt, Mesopotamia, and Crete, were found there only in palaces or in the houses of the rich. The fact that they were so numerous in the Indus cities perhaps means that bathing had not only a hygienic but also a ritual purpose.

The four Vedas are our chief sources of archaic Indian culture and medicine after the Aryan invasion. The word "Veda" means knowledge or sacred lore, and the Vedas were thought to be revealed by the godhead, Brahma, and received by inspired sages who passed them on orally. The text consists of hymns, prayers, incantations, chants, and ritual formulas. Vedic medicine was archaic medicine, and as such, it was very similar to that of other early civilizations, combining religious, magical, and empirical views and practices. The gods were thought to make a mortal sick as a punishment, either directly or through the intermediary of demons; treatment consisted of placating the irate god and driving out and fighting the demons. In addition, a man could become ill as a result of witchcraft, and a disease caused by magic had to be eliminated by magic. Finally, the Indians had a considerable knowledge of drugs and other rational treatments. The administration of these drugs would be accompanied by various incantations.

Although the diseases mentioned in the Vedic books are numerous, they are not described in detail because of the religious nature of the books. Fever, diarrhea, and jaundice are described frequently, as are heart disease and dropsy. Cough is probably a symptom of bronchitis or pneumonia, while consumption is the end stage of a disease that could be, among other things, tuberculosis or cancer. Eye and skin diseases attracted a great deal of attention, and tumors, abscesses, retention of urine, excessive discharges from the body, snake poisoning, and worms, as well as paralysis and mania, are objects of incantations. Like all archaic medicine, it also had empirical and rational elements, probably many more than we can ascertain because we have no medical books from that period. The classical medical literature was the outgrowth of an old tradition, and there can be no doubt that much of its factual content could be traced back to the Vedic period. Medicine was not practiced by priests exclusively but also by laymen who knew symptoms of disease, had knowledge of drugs, and were able to perform certain operations.

In the Brahminical Period (800 B.C.–A.D. 1000), medicine was entirely in the hands of the Brahmin priests and scholars, and the center of medical education was at Benares. There are records showing the existence of hospitals in India before 200 B.C. and in Ceylon in 437 B.C. and in 137 B.C. The ancient Hindus excelled in operative surgery; they amputated limbs, checking hemorrhage by cauterization, boiling oil, or pressure. They treated fractures and dislocations by a special splint made of bamboo. They performed lithotomies, cesarean sections, excisions of tumors, and removed omental hernias through the scrotum. They were particularly skilled in skin grafting and other phases of plastic surgery. It is also noteworthy that their knowledge of infant hygiene and nutrition was unexcelled by any other people until the classical time of the Greeks.

India had early medical schools before and at the time of Buddha; "schools" is here translated as teachers and their disciples, not institutions and buildings. There was a great body of Indian medical writing, of the same nature as the Hippocratic writing, but this cannot be dated with any degree of accuracy. The name of Atreya occurs again and again as being a great physician and medical teacher. The fact that Indian medicine spread to neighboring countries with Buddhism indicates that there was a rational form of medicine as well as magicoreligious medicine at the time of Buddhism. The great Indian epics contain as many references to health, disease, and treatment as do the Homeric poems.

2

Hellenic Medicine

ARCHAIC MEDICINE IN GREECE

UNFORTUNATELY, we have no written documents from the beginnings of Greek medicine, and archaeology only tells us that the palace at Mycenae had bathrooms, toilets, and a drainage system. The Homeric epics are the oldest Greek literature preserved, and we must rely on the *Iliad* and the *Odyssey,* compiled in the ninth and eighth centuries B.C., for our early medical references.

In Greece, as in all ancient civilizations, physiological speculation began with the elementary observation that life is bound to the presence of certain substances of the outside world, such as air and food, and juices of the human body, such as blood. The ancient Egyptians developed the theory that a series of canals connected all parts of the body and carried various substances to and from the organs. The Greeks of Homer's time assumed a relation between food and blood and also recognized the necessity for air. Life was an airlike substance that was breathed out and flew off at the moment of death.

Homeric anatomy, as that of other ancient civilizations, was derived from observations in the kitchen, on the sacrificial altar, and on the battlefield. The chief organs were known, but the early Greeks had only elementary knowledge of their functions. While magical practices survived in uneducated groups or assumed the character of superstition, the empirical and rational components of medicine developed in the schools of the early philosophers and physicians.

It would be unjust to compare the treatment of psychological ailments in ancient Greece with modern methods, for the treatment of

21

mental illness has only recently been put on a scientific basis; in fact, right into the present century mental illness was regarded as a divine affliction, one that could be cured in all sorts of irrational, nonmedical ways. However, although some of the cures claimed are quite fantastic, it is no accident that of the seventy cases listed on the Epidaurian tablets, eleven were cases of blindness, two of deafness, one patient had become voiceless, nine were paralyzed in some part of their bodies, one had insomnia as a result of headaches, and four were of barren women who afterward conceived.

PRE-SOCRATIC PHILOSOPHERS AND EARLY MEDICAL SCHOOLS

Because there is no pre-Hippocratic medical literature on the status of medicine before the end of the sixth century B.C., it does not mean that there was none. The earliest philosophers had no direct influence on medical thought; their primary interest was not in man but in nature and the universe at large. They must be mentioned, however, because their approach to the problems of nature provided a method that was successfully used in the formation of medical theories. These earliest philosophers took nothing for granted but reflected on the nature of things. Everything has a cause, and so the world must have a cause too. Their explanations, although speculative, were rational, and their reasoning was based on careful observations of nature and on a wide range of personal experiences.

Of the early philosophical schools, that of Pythagoras undoubtedly exerted the greatest influence on medicine. The significance of Pythagorean doctrines on medicine is easily apparent. Health is a condition of perfect equilibrium, and the Pythagorean way of life was meant to preserve this equilibrium. By practicing moderation and maintaining equanimity in every situation, an ideal hygienic mode of living was established. If the balance of health has been upset, it must be restored, and the psychosomatic approach of the Pythagoreans, the use of diet, as well as of music, were full of promise. Many pathological processes develop in ways that may be expressed in figures. Malaria is quotidian, tertian, or quartan, that is, the patient has an actue attack of fever every day, or every third or fourth day. Pneumonia and other diseases had crises after certain biologically determined periods. Finally, Pythagorean ideals exerted a strong influence on medical ethics. There is now almost incontestable evidence that the Hippocratic Oath, as it is called, was in fact a Pythagorean document.

Medicine, like mathematics and music, was a field of investigation for the followers of Pythagoras. Philolaus, who lived in the latter half of the fifth century B.C. and who was supposedly the first to write about the teachings of the master, discussed matters of physiology. "The brain is the seat of the mind, the heart of the soul and sensation, the navel of the rooting and growth of the embryo, the genital organ of the emission of sperm and of procreation. The brain signifies the principal of man, the heart that of the animal, the navel that of the plant, the genital organ that of all of them, for they all sprout and grow from sperm."

Medical schools developed in the last third of the sixth century; there were schools not only in Croton but also in Cyrene, Sicily, Rhodes, Cnidus, and Cos. These were not schools of philosophers but of physicians, providing associations of teachers and students, of practitioners and apprentices, many of whom worked as itinerants, carrying with them the tools of their craft—instruments, appliances, drugs —and practicing internal medicine as well as surgery. Their number could not have been large but must have been increasing, for competition became stiff. They are epitomized by Democedes, from the highly regarded school at Croton, who was employed by several states and then became physician to Darius, king of Persia.

Another physician of Croton was Alcmaeon, a philosopher, and although not a Pythagorean, he must have profitted from relationships with members of the school. Like many philosophers, Alcmaeon was interested in problems of physiology, but unlike other philosophers, he dissected animals and performed some simple experiments. He dissected the eye and found it to be connected to the brain by "light-bearing paths." He described these paths as coming together behind the forehead, where they united, and upon this based his explanation as to why both eyes always move together. He also noted that the ears were similarly connected with the brain and surmised that hearing was related to the resonance in these hollow areas. He understood that smell entered the nose with the air and was transmitted to the brain and that the tongue distinguished flavors, although his reasoning here was that, because the tongue was wet, soft, and hot, it melted flavors and separated them according to their looseness of texture and tenderness. He believed that all sense organs were connected with the brain, the seat of sense perception, and that all sensations came together in the brain and were somehow fitted together and stored up so that the brain was also the seat of memory and the organ of thought.

At the time, Alcmaeon was opposed by Aristotle and many other philosophers who believed that the heart was the center of nervous functions. Alcmaeon also opened birds' eggs to watch the embryos, and he believed that the head developed first, rather than the heart as Aristotle believed. Like Pythagoras, he believed that health was a condition of perfect equilibrium between the qualities or forces that are active in the body. He was free from the mysticism of Pythagoras and modest in his awareness of the limitations of science.

LIFE IN THE GREEK CITY-STATES

Athens was not the only cultural center of Greece in the fifth century B.C., and strangely enough, it never developed as a center of medical education. The great medical schools continued to be situated around the periphery of the area of Greek influence. Athens was a polis, like all other Greek city-states, but was also the capital of an empire. Athens set the style for Greek life and was imitated by other city-states. Long after Greece had lost its liberty, the whole of the Western world looked to Athens as the center of culture. This meant, among other things, that the great emphasis put upon health by the Athenians, citizen, metic, or slave, was adopted by the rest of the civilized world. We should, therefore, look at the daily social life of Athens from the point of view of public and personal health.

It was believed that both man and woman secrete semen, and when the two mix in sexual intercourse and the semen is kept in the womb, then pregnancy resulted. If the wife did not conceive, there was supposed to be some good reason for this. The opening of the uterus might be deviated or closed altogether, or it might be slippery by nature or as a result of ulceration. Again, the uterus might be too large or contain residual menstrual blood, or the menstrual flow might be too weak, too strong, or missing altogether; or the uterus might have prolapsed or anteflexed. Many of these explanations are still valid today, but the important thing to note is that infertility was not as-cribed to witchcraft or to the wrath of the gods but was considered the result of natural causes and had to be treated by rational means, such as ointments, fumigations, manipulations, and other measures. Contraceptive devices were employed, and abortions were frequently performed. Abortive drugs were given as potions or pessaries, but as they had no effect whatever, there is no point in listing them. However, certain manipulations, such as the puncture of the conceptus, were more effective.

Plato and Aristotle both recommended abortion as a means of controlling the growth of the population. In his inquiry about the ideal state, Plato suggested that women after the age of forty should be allowed to have intercourse but should not give birth to children; in other words, they should have abortions. Aristotle thought that abortion should be practiced before the embryo had "sensation and life." However, because the Hippocratic Oath forbids the physician to "give to a woman an abortive pessary," it seems difficult to reconcile this prohibition with the facts that abortion was generally practiced, not only by midwives but also by Hippocratic and other physicians, that it was accepted by society, and that it was even recommended by the greatest philosophers of the period. The average Greek did not have the deep respect for life that the Indian had. Weak and crippled infants were destroyed, not only in Sparta but also in Athens; and once one is prepared to kill born children, why should there be any hesitation to destroy a mere embryo, provided it can be done without endangering the mother? There were, however, religious groups in Greek society, notably the Orphics and Pythagoreans, who, perhaps under Indian influence, had a profound respect for life. We have noted that the so-called Hippocratic Oath was actually a Pythagorean document, which therefore, did not represent the general view of the period but was rather a reform program, a manifesto of a relatively small religious group.

Athenian education was aimed at developing the whole man, both physical and mental. This ideal had great hygienic value because general education and health education went hand in hand. The physician had as his close allies the educator and the physical trainer. In any civilization, the success or failure of health education depends not only on the knowledge of the physician but also on society's willingness to accept advice. Where health is highly valued and people consider it their duty to maintain a healthy body, then the physician has no trouble in having his advice accepted. Health knowledge did not all flow from the physician. He also received help from the educators or philosophers and the trainers. The trainers were keen observers, knew quite a lot about surface anatomy, and were able to give advice on the correct diet (in the Greek sense), which would provide for the best physical and mental well-being. The Hippocratic collection contains two treatises on diet that were written both for the physician and the layman.

HIPPOCRATIC MEDICINE

Hippocrates is believed to have been born on the island of Cos in about 460 B.C. and to have lived until about 370 B.C. Although no other physician has achieved greater fame, we actually know very little about him. The only contemporary references are in two dialogues of Plato. From these, we learn that Hippocrates was a teacher of medicine who accepted students upon payment of a tuition fee and that he was so well known everybody knew about him. Because all his biographies are posthumous, however, they are open to doubt.

Hippocrates is justly eminent on three accounts; first, he disassociated medicine from the supernatural and from philosophy; second, he crystalized the loose knowledge of the Coan and Cnidian schools into a systematic science; and third, he gave physicians the highest moral inspiration that they have ever had. In the words of Edelstein: "Hippocrates considered the body an organism; medical practice he based on the knowledge resulting from the comprehension of the scattered particulars into one concept and the division of the whole in turn into its natural species."

There are numerous so-called Hippocratic writings, but there is considerable doubt as to which of them, if any, were actually written by Hippocrates; however, the ideas expressed in these writings are attributed to him. He appears to be the founder of scientific medicine, basing his actions upon observation and reasoning. Until very recently, his theories, particularly after having been systematized by Galen, were the dominating influence in the development of Western medicine. Anatomy receives scant treatment in the Hippocratic writings. It is primitive and, in a way, speculative, but it does indicate that the systematic dissection of animals was carried out. There is also a considerable number of theoretical writings that are very different in both style and content. Although the treatise "On Ancient Medicine" is written in a philosophical vein, it points out that medicine is an art that originated empirically after it was found that certain foods and diets improved the condition of sick people, and it deplores the intrusion of philosophy into medicine. The treatise "On the Nature of Man" seems to be one of the later writings of the collection, and its importance lies in the fact that it describes the theory of the four humors (blood, phlegm, yellow bile, and black bile) that was to dominate medicine for many centuries in both East and West. Drugs are mentioned in a great many books, but pharmacological therapy does not play an important part in Hippocratic medicine. Its drugs were mostly household remedies.

THE HIPPOCRATIC PHYSICIAN

The time of Hippocrates was a rational age that was not satisfied with ascribing disease to the wrath of the gods. In earlier civilizations, it was believed that disease was the punishment for sin sent from the gods. The Greeks believed in all sorts of punishments sent from the gods, but disease was not one of them. The Greek world of the classical age was for the healthy and the sound; illness in Greece carried the burden of inferiority. The Greek ideal of culture was one of physical and mental development and well-being. The sick, the crippled, the weakling were inferior and may count on society's attention only if their condition improved. This attitude obviously had a considerable effect upon the standing of the physician in the community. As a man who worked for money and practiced a craft, he would not have held a very high social position, but the importance of health in the community meant that he was not treated as other craftsmen, particularly if he were renowned. In addition, medicine was more than a craft, for it incorporated a philosophy. For this reason, many educated Greeks engaged in medical studies without ever intending to practice as physicians.

The young man who wanted to study medicine and practice as a physician became an apprentice. He paid a fee and worked with a physician for a number of years, seeing patients with him, assisting him in preparing remedies and performing operations, keeping his surgery in order, listening to the oral instructions of the master, and making notes of what he saw and heard. Using only a good open mind and keen perception, Hippocrates demonstrated the high standard of practice that internal medicine could attain. Medicine owes to him the art of clinical inspection and observation. His honesty and integrity were such that he felt a constant obligation to provide each patient with the very best care, and he felt an equally heavy responsibility to maintain the highest ethical and moral standards. Hippocrates really instituted the bedside method of patient care and the bedside method of student teaching. Because of this, his students were exposed to the highest standards of medical practice and the highest standards of personal behavior.

The foundation of medical ethics is generally acknowledged to be the Hippocratic Oath, which is as follows:

I swear by Apollo physician and Asclepius and Hygieia and Panaceia and all the gods and goddesses, making them my witnesses, that I will fulfill according to my ability and judgement this oath and this covenant:

To hold him who has taught me this art as equal to my parents and to live my life in partnership with him, and if he is in need of money to give him a share of mine, and to regard his offspring as my brothers in male lineage and to teach them this art—if they desire to learn it—without fee or covenant; to give a share of precepts and oral instruction and all the other learning to my sons and to the sons of him who has instructed me and to pupils who have signed the covenant and have taken an oath according to the medical law, but to no one else.

I will apply dietetic measures for the benefit of the sick according to my ability and judgement; I will keep them from harm and injustice.

I will neither give a deadly drug to anybody if asked for it, nor will I make a suggestion to this effect.

Similarly I will not give to a woman an abortive remedy.

In purity and holiness I will guard my life and my art.

I will not use the knife, not even on sufferers from stone, but will withdraw in favor of such men as are engaged in this work.

Whatever houses I may visit, I will come for the benefit of the sick, remaining free of all intentional injustice, of all mischief, and in particular of sexual relations with both female and male persons, be they free or slaves.

What I may see or hear in the course of the treatment or even outside of the treatment in regard to the life of men, which on no account one must noise abroad, I will keep to myself, holding such things shameful to be spoken about.

If I fulfill this oath and do not violate it, may it be granted to me to enjoy life and art, being honored with fame among all men for all time to come; if I transgress it and swear falsely, may the opposite of all this be my lot.

The oath naturally divides into two parts: the first dealing with the relationship between the physician and his pupil and the second dealing with the relationship between the physician and the patient. It is customary to consider only the second part, that is, the relationship with patients, to be concerned with ethics, but when one studies the oath carefully, it becomes apparent that the whole document is concerned with ethical considerations.

The evidence indicates that the Hippocratic covenant was inspired by Pythagorean doctrine and was later adopted by physicians in respect to the acceptance of pupils. Over the centuries, there has been a much-decreased emphasis placed on the physician's obligations to his pupils. It is now customary to regard only that part of the oath that deals with the physician's relationship to his patients as having any ethical impact today. The Code of Ethics of the American Medical Association and its subsequent revisions have been based upon the Hippocratic Oath but have ignored the physician's obligations in the field of medical education completely.

The second half of the oath is concerned with the ethical standards that should guide a physician in his relationship with a patient and the patient's family. Careful investigation of the medical and ethical stipulations, particularly the inflexible provisions concerning the application of poisons and of abortive remedies, indicates that the second part of the oath is influenced by Pythagorean ideas. The physician is asked to use dietetic means to the advantage of his patients as his judgment and capacity permit, but he also is asked to go beyond this and keep his patients from mischief and injustice. It is obvious that the doctor's dietetic prescriptions should be given to help the patient, and every ancient physician would have subscribed to this idea. Pythagorean physicians did not feel any differently.

However, the distinctly Pythagorean influence is seen in the physician's promise to guard his patients against the evils that they may suffer through themselves. It was a Pythagorean belief that man is naturally liable to inflict upon himself injustice and mischief, particularly in his day-to-day living. The Pythagoreans believed that all bodily appetites were cravings of the soul for the presence or absence of certain things. They believed that the body should take in a certain amount of food and should be cleansed again appropriately after it has been filled. The physician felt that he had a duty to advise the healthy along these lines, and of course, he would feel an added obligation to the sick person whom he was treating. This is the most likely reason for the physician to feel he must protect his patient from the mischief and injustice that he might inflict upon himself if his diet were not properly chosen.

The next section of the oath reads: "I will neither give a deadly drug to anybody if asked for it, nor will I make a suggestion to this effect. Similarly I will not give to a woman an abortive remedy." If a sick Greek felt that his pains had become intolerable, if no help could be expected, he would often put an end to his own life. The taking of poison was the most usual way of committing suicide, and the patient was likely to demand the poison from his physician, who was in possession of deadly drugs and knew which ones brought about an easy and painless end. The resolve to commit suicide would not be taken without due deliberation, and the sick person would wish to be sure that further treatment would be of no avail. He or his friends would therefore consult the physician. Thus, it is unlikely that the interdiction of poison and of abortive remedies was simply the outgrowth of medical ethics. It would appear, then, that this part of the oath was governed by a philosophical conviction, and this view is enhanced by the next statement in the oath: "In purity and holiness I will guard my life and my art." If men decided to take their lives, they were within their rights as sovereign masters of themselves. Among all the Greek thinkers, only the Pythagoreans completely outlawed suicide. This school was absolutely opposed to suicide and believed it was a sin against the gods, who had allocated to man his position in life as a post to be held and defended.

The ancient practitioner was a surgeon as well as a physician, and therefore, it is nonsense to suggest that the forswearing of the use of the knife in the next part of the oath is intended to draw a line between the practice of internal medicine and the practice of surgery. There is evidence from Aristoxenes and Plato that the Pythagoreans refused to apply any surgical means of treatment. This is a logical outcome of their belief that the shedding of blood was a defilement. If we believe the oath to be a Pythagorean document, this vow not to use the knife makes sense, and it also makes sense that the person who swore the oath went on to say "but will withdraw in favor of such men as are engaged in this work."

The rest of the oath is concerned with ethical standards that were higher than the average behavior of the times but that agreed with Pythagorean beliefs. Gradually, the ethics of the medical profession with regard both to behavior in the patient's house and to professional silence have been raised to reach the level first set by Pythagoras and his followers.

ARISTOTLE

Aristotle gave to medicine the beginnings of botany, zoology, comparative anatomy, embryology, teratology, and physiology. Although the Greeks did not practice human dissection, Aristotle dissected animals and used them in the teaching of anatomy. He was a pupil of Plato and developed the use of formal logic as an instrument of precision. However, he surpassed Plato in the direct observation of external nature and was so great an experimental researcher that he deserves his place as one of the greatest biologists of all times. His doctrine of the primacy of the heart as the source of "innate heat" and as the seat of sensation and thought makes him very weak in the field of physiology, but unfortunately, for two thousand years he was considered so infallible that his judgments could not be challenged, and his misconceptions persisted to the disadvantage of medical progress.

In the following extract, from *Parts of Animals,* Aristotle discusses the generative process and the relation of structure to function:

Now there are three degrees of composition; and of these the first in order, as all will allow, is composition out of what some call the elements, such as earth, air, water, fire. Perhaps, however, it would be more accurate to say composition out of the elementary forces; nor indeed out of all of these, but out of a limited number of them, as defined in previous treatises. For fluid and solid, hot and cold, form the material of all composite bodies; and all other differences are secondary to these such differences, that is, as heaviness or lightness, density or rarity, roughness or smoothness, and any other such properties of matter as there may be. The second degree of composition is that by which the homogeneous parts of animals, such as bone, flesh, and the like, are constituted out of the primary substances. The third and last stage is the composition which forms the heterogeneous parts, such as face, hand, and the rest.

Now the order of actual development and the order of logical existence are always the inverse of each other. For that which is posterior in the order of development is antecedent in the order of nature, and that is genetically last which in nature is first.

(That this is so is manifest by induction; for a house does not exist for the sake of bricks and stones, but these materials for the sake of the house; and the same is the case with the materials of other bodies. Nor is induction required to show this. It is included in our conception of generation. For generation is a process from a something to a something; that which is generated having a cause in which it originates and a cause in which it ends. The originating cause is the primary efficient cause, which is something already endowed with tangible existence, while the final cause is some definite form or similar end; for man generates man, and plant generates plant, in each case out of the underlying material.)

In order of time, then, the material and the generative process must necessarily be anterior to the being that is generated; but in logical order the definitive character and form of each being precedes the material. This is evident if one only tries to define the process of formation. For the definition of house-building includes and presupposes that of the house; but the definition of the house does not include nor presuppose that of house-building; and the same is true of all other productions. So that it must necessarily be that the elementary material exists for the sake of the homogeneous parts, seeing that these are genetically posterior to it, just as the heterogeneous parts are posterior genetically to them. For these heterogeneous parts have reached the end and goal, having the third degree of composition, in which degree generation or development often attains its final term.

Animals, then, are composed of homogeneous parts, and are also composed of heterogeneous parts. The former, however, exist for the sake of the latter. For the active functions and operations of the body are carried on by these; that is, by the heterogeneous parts, such as the eye, the nostril, the whole face, the fingers, the hand, and the whole arm. But inasmuch as there is a great variety in the functions and motions not only of aggregate animals but also of the individual organs, it is necessary that the substances out of which these are composed shall present a diversity of properties. For some purposes softness is advantageous, for others hardness; some parts must be capable of extension, others of flexion. Such properties, then, are distributed separately to the different homogeneous parts, one being soft another hard, one fluid another solid, one viscous another brittle; whereas each of the heterogeneous parts presents a combination of multifarious properties. For the hand, to take an example, requires one property to enable it to effect pressure, and a different property for simple prehension. For this reason the active or executive parts of the body are compounded out of bones, sinews, flesh, and the like, but not these latter out of the former.

So far, then, as has yet been stated, the relations between these two orders of parts are determined by a final cause. We have, however, to inquire whether necessity may not also have a share in the matter; and it must be admitted that these mutual relations could not from the very beginning have possibly been other than they are. For heterogeneous parts can be made up out of homogeneous parts, either from a plurality of them, or from a single one, as is the case with some of the viscera which, varying in configuration, are yet, to speak broadly, formed from a single homogeneous substance; but that homogeneous substances should be formed out of a combination of heterogeneous parts is clearly an impossibility. For these causes, then, some parts of animals are simple and homogeneous, while others are composite and heterogeneous; and dividing the parts into the active or exactive and the sensitive, each one of the former is, as before said, heterogeneous, and each one of the latter homogeneous. For it is in homogeneous parts alone that sensation can occur, as the following considerations show.

Each sense is confined to a single order of sensibles, and its organ must be such as to admit the action of that kind of order. But it is only that which is endowed with a property *in posse* [in potency] that is acted on by that which has the like property *in esse* [in existence], so that the two are the same in kind, and if the latter is single or so also is the former. Thus it is that while no physiologists ever dream of saying of the hand or face or other such part that one is earth, another water, another fire, they couple each separate sense-organ with a separate element, asserting this one to be air and that other to be fire.

Sensation, then, is confined to the simple or homogeneous parts. But, as might reasonably be expected, the organ of touch, though still homogeneous, is yet the least simple of all the sense-organs. For touch more than any other sense appears to be correlated to several distinct kinds of objects, and to recognize more than one category of contrasts, heat and cold, for instance, solidity and fluidity, and other similar oppositions. Accordingly, the organ which deals with these varied objects is of all the sense-organs the most corporeal, being either the flesh, or the substance which in some animals takes the place of flesh.

Now as there cannot possibly be an animal without sensation, it follows as a necessary consequence that every animal must have some homogeneous parts; for these alone are capable of sensation, the heterogeneous parts serving for the active functions. Again, as the sensory faculty, the motor faculty, and the nutritive faculty are all lodged in one and the same part of the body, as was stated in a former treatise, it is necessary that the part which is the primary seat of these principles shall on the one hand, in its character of general sensory recipient, be one of the simple parts; and on the other hand shall, in its motor and active character, be one of the heterogeneous parts. For this reason it is the heart which in sanguineous animals constitutes this central part, and in bloodless animals it is that which takes the place of a heart. For the heart, like the other viscera, is one of the homogeneous parts; for, if cut up, its pieces are homogeneous in substance with each other. But it is at the same time heterogeneous in virtue of its definite configuration. And the same is true of the other so-called viscera, which are indeed formed from the same material as the heart. For all these viscera have a sanguineous character owing to their being situated upon vascular ducts and branches. For just as a stream of water deposits mud, so the various viscera, the heart excepted, are, as it were, deposits from the stream of blood in the vessels. And as to the heart, the very starting-point of the vessels, and the actual seat of the force by which the blood is first fabricated, it is but what one would naturally expect, that out of the selfsame nutriment of which it is the recipient its own proper substance shall be formed. Such, then, are the reasons why the viscera are of sanguineous aspect; and why in one point of view they are homogeneous, in another heterogeneous. (*De Partibus Animalium*, Lib. III, Cap. I)

3

Hellenistic Medicine

DURING THE nineteenth century, German historian Gustav Droysen (1808–84) introduced a new concept into the traditional practice of dividing ancient history into separate Greek and Roman epochs. As a result of the conquests of Alexander the Great, he taught, a new political amalgam evolved that was not based on "national" societies but on the universalism of the idea of the *oecumene,* or "inhabited world," where all men lived as brothers. From the Indus in the East to the Rhine in the West, there was a diffusion of common cultural elements. In art, architecture, education, and life-style, a degree of sophistication was achieved that would not be surpassed until modern times.

As far as medicine was concerned, this era ushered in changes that were to dominate until the scientific revolution of the seventeenth century. Perhaps the most important change was the professionalization of medicine. The urbanization of large segments of the population necessitated the creation of a more professional corps to deal with the problems of hygiene and disease. Hence, one of the most important contributions of the Hellenistic age was the maintenance of salaried public physicians.

Although the earlier Greeks had occasionally employed physicians, the post-Alexandrian world introduced the practice of supporting salaried public doctors. By the first century after the Christian era, almost every large city in the empire possessed a number of official doctors. Their chief responsibility was to give medical aid to the citizens, and although allowed to accept fees, they were required to care for those who could not pay. Additional duties included certify-

35

ing the cause of death in cases of suspected homicide and examining injuries in court cases involving assault. In addition, the Egyptian practice of embalming broke down the Greek reluctance to dissect the human body, thereby ushering in a new era in the study of anatomy.

Alexandria, founded in 332 B.C. by the conqueror whose name it bears, was the great metropolis of the Hellenistic world. Its library and museum, founded by Ptolemy I, housed the treasures of the civilized world. The library contained almost half a million rolls of papyri; the finest scholars, artists, scientists, and poets of the age gathered there. Its school of medicine was to remain the center of medical studies for the next three centuries. Long after the conquest of Egypt by the Romans in 31 B.C., Alexandria dominated the intellectual and cultural world.

Herophilus of Chalcedon-Bithynia was among the earlier famous physicians of the school of Alexandria. Some regard Herophilus as one of the founders of anatomy. His studies of the brain and the spinal cord and his insistence that the brain was the central organ of the nervous system and of intelligence brought him into conflict with the Aristotelians, who thought the heart was the organ of intelligence. He was the first to distinguish between the cerebellum and the cerebrum and to divide the nerves into sensory and motor. His description of the abdominal organs included the liver, pancreas, and duodenum, which he named. Herophilus made the first clear distinction between the arteries and veins and counted the pulse by means of a water clock. Because of his studies of pulse rate and his scientific observation of systole and diastole, he is regarded as the father of cardiology.

Erasistratus of Chios was associated with Herophilus at Alexandria. Trained in the school of Cnidos, he brought to Alexandria the long tradition of its Indian and Persian contacts. Unlike Herophilus, he rejected the humoral theory of Hippocrates and ascribed the causes of disease to changes in the solids of the body. It was his belief that the veins were the conduits of blood and the arteries carried air. Inhaled air was carried to the heart, where it was transformed into vital spirit, which was then changed in the brain into animal spirit. The latter was then carried to the body by the nervous system. He regarded the brain as the center for all spiritual functions. Unlike many of his contemporaries, he was opposed to bloodletting, which he rejected because of the problems of finding the vein, of erroneously opening the artery, and determining the quantity of blood to be taken.

It is recorded that both Herophilus and Erasistratus practiced vivisection on human beings.

Herophilus and Erasistratus synthesized the rival traditions of Cos and Cnidos, the former with its emphasis on the overall disease, the latter with its focus on the symptoms found in the patient. Both founded schools that lasted for over a century and that included among their followers many of the distinguished physicians of the first century of the Christian era.

Toward the end of the third century, a new medical tradition developed in Alexandria. Termed empiricism, it was basically a revolt against the overspeculative aspects of Greek medicine. It stood in opposition to the so-called Rational School that treated disease according to determined rules. The founder of the Empiricists, Philinus of Cos, broke with the Herophilean School because he found that it was useless to speculate on the remote causes of disease and that a knowledge of anatomy played no role in treating the sick. For the Empiricists, medicine was simply a matter of therapeutics. Serapion of Alexandria, who rejected all dogmatic teaching on physiology and pathology, was more radical than his contemporary Philinus. For Serapion, all medical practice was based on a trinity of principles; personal experience, experience of others derived through history, and analogy. The most well known of the Empiricists was the Greek-born Heraclides of Taras, who lived during the first century before Christ. His work "On the Preparation of Drugs" was one of the most highly respected works on materia medica until the time of Galen. Among drugs recommended were cinnamon, pepper, and opium. The latter he prescribed for spasms, hydrophobia, cholera, and insomnia. A surgeon as well as a physician, he is said to have invented instruments for reducing dislocations of the hip joint and a mechanical method of separating the lid from the eyeball. By the beginning of the Christian era, Empiricism had degenerated into a sterile form of quackery.

Another school of medicine, called Methodism and identified with Themison of Laodicea (143–123 B.C.), appeared during the Hellenistic period. Themison was a student of Asclepiades of Bithynia, the first physician to establish Hellenic medicine in Rome. Both men rejected much of the Hippocratic tradition, the humoral theory as well as the concept that the physician should not interfere with nature. Asclepiades followed the philosophy of Democritus in viewing disease as a result of disharmonious conditions in the motion of the body.

Unlike Hippocrates, he gave great attention to chronic diseases, and the more urbanized society of the Hellenistic world is contrasted with rural Greece. Themison thought that sickness resulted from clogged pores and from stagnation of small solids caused by the contraction of tissue or the rapid movement of solids caused by the relaxation of the pores. The Methodists claimed that disease should be judged by its symptoms rather than by its cause. Common cures were bloodletting, poultices, diet control, and laxatives. The theory failed to provide for the treatment of surgical conditions, fractures, tumors, and so on. Yet it was considered a step beyond the blind adulation of the Hippocratics and the Empiricists, limited as they were to self-experience. Perhaps the best-known physician of the Methodist School was Soranus of Ephesus (98–138). Because of his work *Diseases of Women* and his studies of female anatomy, Soranus is regarded as the greatest gynecologist and obstetrician of the Hellenistic world. He was one of the first physicians to note that the human uterus was not convoluted as in animals. His description of the use of the obstetrical chair and the vaginal speculum place him centuries ahead of his contemporaries. The first part of the *Diseases of Women* covers such subjects as the stages of conception, pregnancy, and delivery as well as means of birth control. In the second section, he discusses such female complaints as amenorrhea, dysmenorrhea, condylomata, and gonorrhea. Soranus' work *On Acute and Chronic Diseases* has come down to us in the Latin version of African-born Caelus Aurelianus, who, like Soranus, was a member of the Methodist School. The work was first printed in the sixteenth century; in the following selection, the problem of homosexuality is discussed:

People find it hard to believe that effeminate men or pathetics really exist. The fact is that, though the practices of such persons are unnatural to human beings, lust overcomes modesty and puts to shameful use parts intended for other functions. That is, in the case of certain individuals, there is no limit to their desire and no hope of satisfying it; and they cannot be content with their own lot, the lot which divine providence has marked out for them in assigning definite functions to the parts of the body. They even adopt the dress, walk, and other characteristics of women. Now this condition is different from a bodily disease; it is rather an affliction of a diseased mind. Indeed, often out of passion and in rare cases out of respect for certain persons to whom they are indebted, these pathetics suddenly change their character and for a time try to give proof of their virility. But since they are not aware of their limitations, they are again the victims of excesses, subjecting their virility to too great a strain and consequently involving themselves in worse vices. And it is our opinion that these persons suffer no impairment of sensation. For, as Soranus says, this affliction comes from a corrupt and debased mind. Indeed, the victims of this malady may be compared to the women who are called *tribades* because they pursue both kinds of love. These women are more eager to lie with women than men; in fact, they pursue women with almost masculine jealousy, and when they are freed or temporarily relieved of their passion . . . they rush, as if victims of continual intoxication, to new forms of lust, and, sustained by this disgraceful mode of life, they rejoice in the abuse of their sexual powers. So the pathetics, like the *tribades,* are victims of an affliction of the mind. For there exists no bodily treatment which can be applied to overcome the disease; it is rather the mind that is affected in these disgraceful vices, and it is consequently the mind which must be controlled. For no man has ever overcome bodily lust by playing the woman's sexual role, or gained relief by contact with the penis. In general, the relief of pain and disease is achieved by other means. Thus the account of a cure as given by Clodius obviously refers to a case of ascarides. The latter, as we showed in our chapter on worms, are small worms arising in the parts of the rectum.

Parmenides in his work *On Nature* indicates that effeminate men or pathetics may come into being as the result of a circumstance at conception. Since his account is contained in a Greek poem, I shall also give my version in poetry. For I have done my best to compose Latin verses of the same kind, to avoid the commingling of the two languages.

"When man and woman mingle the seeds of love that spring from their veins, a formative power maintaining proper proportions molds well-formed bodies from this diverse blood. For if, when the seed is mingled, the forces contained therein clash and do not fuse into one, then cruelly will they plague with double seed the sex of the offspring."

Thus Parmenides holds that the seminal fluids are not merely material bodies but possess active principles, and if these fluids mingle in such a way as to form a unified force in the body, they will thereby produce a desire appropriate to the sex of the individual. But if, despite the mingling of the seminal matter, the active principles fail to merge, a desire for both forms of love will harass the offspring.

On the other hand, many leaders of the other sects hold that the condition which we are discussing is an inherited disease, that is to say, passed on from generation to generation by way of the seed. For this they do not blame nature, since the latter shows its strict purity by the example of the brute animals, whom philosophers call "nature's mirrors." These physicians place the blame rather on the human race, because, having once incurred the defects, it retains them and cannot rid itself of them by any kind of renovation, and leaves no opportunity for a fresh start . . . though other diseases, whether hereditary or adventitious, in the great majority of cases become weaker as the body grows older; this is true, for example, of podagra, epilepsy, and mania, which unquestionably become milder in the patient's declining years. The fact is that whatever irritates will produce its strongest effect when the underlying matter offers strong opposition; but, since such opposition fades in the case of old people, disease, like strength is also blunted. But the affliction under discussion, which produces effeminate men or pathetics, is the only one that becomes stronger as the body grows older. It causes a hideous and ever increasing lust. And there is good reason why this takes place. For in other years when the body is still strong and can perform the normal functions of love, the sexual desire [of these persons] assumes a dual aspect, in which the soul is excited sometimes while playing a passive role and sometimes while playing an active role. But in the cases of old men who have lost their virile powers, all their sexual desire is turned in the opposite direction and consequently exerts a stronger demand for the feminine role in love. In fact, many infer that this is the reason why boys too are victims of this affliction. For, like old men, they do not possess virile powers; that is, they have not yet attained those powers which have already deserted the aged. (*Caeli Aureliani Methodici Siccensis Tardarum Passionum,* Lib. IV, Cap. IX)

The Hellenistic world was divided along philosophical lines, and it must be recalled that medicine was at that time considered a branch of philosophy. Three distinct schools had emerged by the third century B.C., and while they did not affect medicine directly, their views of humanity reflect the society in which the physician performed his tasks.

The Cynics, founded by Antisthenes of Athens, a disciple of Socrates, were so called because they resembled dogs, *Kines,* in their disregard for convention. As a group, the Cynics opposed all culture except insofar as it produced virtue. Unlike Socrates, who said virtue is good, the Cynic said that virtue is the only good and vice the only evil. Aside from virtue, nothing—riches, honors, freedom, health, even death—has true value. For the Cynic, the essence of virtue is self-control and independence from all material things. In a sense, it was an escapist philosophy, a kind of primitivism that advocated the abolition of all civic and social ties and all restrictions except those that arise out of a sense of duty. Characterized by a sort of ostentatious asceticism, it demonstrated traits later seen in Manichaeism, the mendicant movement of the Middle Ages, and the current fad of escapism found among the hippies.

The Cynic School was eventually absorbed by that of the more reasonable Stoics. Like the Cynics, the Stoics traced their doctrines back to Socrates, although there was a dependence upon the ideas of Heraclitus and Aristotle. Zeno, a native of Cyprus who had studied with the Cynics in Athens, is regarded as the founder of the school. The term "Stoic" is derived from the Painted Porch, which was the name of its first school. The Heraclitean belief that all things are in a state of constant flux was basic to the Stoic interpretation of the universe. The Stoics held that the material world alone is real. Whatever distinction there may be between corporeal and incorporeal beings is based upon a mere distinction between coarser and finer matter. They described the human soul as a fiery breath diffused throughout the body. They advocated the unity of the human race, justice in the state, and the equality of men and women. They also exhibited certain elements of Oriental mysticism, including the notions that the wise man is emancipated from all moral law and that the individual must be self-sufficient and independent of all externals. Stoicism had a tremendous effect on Hellenistic Rome, molding its laws and adding an element of humanism to its rigid legal system. Unlike the Cynics, who held the body in disdain, the Stoics respected good physical appearance.

One of the most well known of the Stoic philosophers was the former slave, Epictetus, who resided in Rome during the reigns of Nero and Trajan. In his famous *Discourses,* he explains his attitude toward cleanliness:

Some men raise the question whether the social faculty is a necessary element in man's nature: nevertheless even they, I think, would not question that cleanliness at any rate is essential to it, and that this, if anything, divides him from the lower animals. So when we see one of the other animals cleaning itself, we are wont to say in our surprise, "He does it like a man." And again, if some one finds fault with an animal for being dirty we are wont to say at once, as if in defence, "Of course he is not a man." So true is it that we think the quality to be distinctive of man, deriving it first from the gods. For since the gods are by nature pure and unalloyed, in so far as men have approached them by virtue of reason, they have a tendency to purity and cleanliness. But since it is impossible for their nature to be entirely pure, being composed of such stuff as it is, the reason which they have received endeavours, so far as in it lies, to make this stuff clean.

The primary and fundamental purity is that of the soul, and so with impurity. You cannot find the same impurity in a soul as in a body: the soul's impurity you will find to be just this—that which renders it unclean for its own functions; and the functions of a soul are: impulse to act and not to act, will to get and will to avoid, preparation, design, assent. What is it then which renders the soul foul and unclean in these functions? It is nothing but its evil judgements. And so the soul's impurity consists in bad judgements and purification consists in producing in it right judgements, and the pure soul is one which has right judgements, for this alone is proof against confusion and pollution in its functions.

And one ought to endeavour, as far as may be, to achieve a similar cleanliness in one's body too. Man's temperament is such that there must needs be mucous discharge: for this reason nature made hands, and the nostrils themselves like channels to cleanse his humours. If he swallows them I say that he does not act as a man should. It was impossible for men's feet not to be made muddy and dirty when they pass through mud and dirt; for this reason nature provided water and hands to wash with. It was impossible that some impurity should not stick to the teeth from eating. Therefore we are bidden to wash our teeth. Why: That you may be a man and not a beast or a pig. It was impossible that sweat and the pressure of our clothes should not leave some defilement clinging to the body, and needing to be cleansed. Therefore we have water, olive-oil, hands, towel, strigils, soap, and on occasion every other sort of apparatus, to make the body clean.

"Not for me," you say.

What! The smith will clean his iron tool of rust, and will have instruments made for the purpose, and even you will wash your plate when you are going to eat, unless you are absolutely foul and dirty, and yet you will not wash nor make clean your poor body? "Why should I?" says he. I will tell you again: first, that you may act like a man, next, that you may not annoy those you meet. You are doing something very like it even here, though you are not aware of it. You think you deserve to have a scent of your own. Very well, deserve it: but do you think those who sit by you deserve it too, and those who recline by you, and those who kiss you? Go away then into a wilderness, where you deserve to go, and live by yourself, and have your smell to yourself, for it is right that you should enjoy your uncleanness by yourself; but if you are in a city, what sort of man are you making yourself, to behave so thoughtlessly and inconsiderately? If nature had trusted a horse to your care, would you have left it uncared for? Imagine that your body has been committed to you as a horse: wash it, rub it down well, make it such that no one will shun it or turn from it. But who does not turn from a man who is dirty, odorous, foul-complexioned, more from one who is bespattered with muck? The smell of the latter is external and accidental, that of the former comes from want of tendance; it is from within, and shows a sort of inward rottenness. (*Dissertationes*, Lib. IV, Cap. I)

The founder of the Epicureans, Lucretius of Samos, claimed complete originality in the system he instituted in Athens in the third century. For the Epicurean, the good life consists of the enjoyment of pleasure, but in a negative sense. Happiness is the avoidance of pain, worry, and anxiety. There is a certain hierachy of pleasures, the highest of which are of the mind, knowledge, and intelligence, as they free the soul from prejudice and fear and contribute to its repose. The human soul, which resembles the gods, is composed of finer atoms, air, fire, vapor, and a nameless seat of rationality located in the breast. It is the soul that holds the body together, and death results when the corporeal protection ceases.

Lucretius' "law of diseases" held that an accumulation of adverse factors fouled the air, giving rise to disease. In the following, he enunciates this law and draws attention to the differences of diseases in different climates:

And now I will explain what the law of diseases is and from what causes the force of disease may suddenly gather itself up and bring death-dealing destruction on the race of man and the troops of brute beasts. And first I have shown above that there are seeds of many things helpful to our life; and on the other hand many must fly about conducing to disease and death. When these by chance have happened to gather together and have disordered the atmosphere, the air becomes distempered. And all that force of disease and that pestilence come either from without down through the atmosphere in the shape of clouds and mists, or else do gather themselves up and rise out of the earth, when soaked with wet it has contracted a taint, being beaten upon by unseasonable rains and suns. See you not too that all who come to a place far away from country and home are affected by the strangeness of climate and water, because there are wide differences in such things? For what a difference may we suppose between the climate of the Briton and that of Egypt where the pole of heaven slants askew, and again between that in Pontus and that of Gades and so on to the races of men black with sun-baked complexion? Now as we see these four climates under the four opposite winds and quarters of heaven all differing from each other, so also the complexions and faces of the men are seen to differ widely and diseases varying in kind are found to seize upon the different races. There is the elephant disease which is generated beside the streams of Nile in the midst of Egypt and nowhere else. In Attica the feet are attacked and the eyes in Achaean lands. And so different places are hurtful to different parts and members: the variations of air occasion that. Therefore when an atmosphere which happens to put itself in motion unsuited to us and a hurtful air begin to advance, they creep slowly on in the shape of mist and cloud and disorder everything in their line of advance and compel all to change; and when they have at length reached our atmosphere, they corrupt it too and make it like to themselves and unsuited to us. This new destroying power and pestilence therefore all at once either fall upon the waters or else sink deep into the corncrops or other food of man and provender of beast; or else their force remains suspended within the atmosphere, and when we inhale from it mixed airs, we must absorb at the same time into our body those things as well. In like manner pestilence often falls on kine also and a distemper too on the silly sheep. And it makes no difference whether we travel to places unfavourable to us and change the atmosphere which wraps us round, or whether nature without our choice brings to us a tainted atmosphere or something to the use of which we have not been accustomed, and which is able to attack us on its first arrival. (*De Rerum Natura*, Lib. VI)

We have already said that it is not quite proper to speak of Roman medicine, but rather of Greek medicine in Rome. By the second century B.C., Roman conquests in the eastern Mediterranean had brought them into contact with the brilliant Hellenistic world, and many of the ultraconservatives thought that this culture was a definite threat to the traditional doctrine of subordination of oneself to family, class, state, and gods. Marcus Cato (234–149 B.C.) was chief spokesman of this narrow conservative and nationalistic view. The influx of physicians into Rome was one of the elements of the new culture that he ranted against. From the *Natural History* of Pliny, we have an account of Cato's reaction to change:

Cassius Hemina, one of our most ancient writers, is authority for the statement that the first physician that came to Rome was Archagathus, the son of Lysanias, who came over from the Peloponnesus in the 535th year of the city, in the consulship of Lucius Aemilius and Marcus Livius. He states also that the Roman citizenship was granted him, and that he had a shop provided for his practice at the public expense the Acilian Crossway; that he was a remarkable healer of wounds; that at the beginning his arrival was extraordinarily welcome, but that soon afterwards, from his cruelty in cutting and cauterizing, he acquired the name of Carnifex [executioner], and brought his art and physicians into disrepute.

This may be most clearly understood from the words of Marcus Cato, whose authority does not need to be bolstered by his triumph and censorship —so high does it rank of itself. I shall, therefore, cite his own words: "Concerning those Greeks, son Marcus, I will speak to you in the proper place. I will show you the results of my own experience at Athens: that it is a good idea to dip into their literature but not to learn it thoroughly. I shall convince you that they are a most iniquitous and intractable people, and you may take my word as the word of a prophet: whenever that nation shall bestow its literature upon us, it will corrupt everything, and all the sooner if it sends its physicians here. They have conspired among themselves to murder all foreigners with their medicine, a profession which they exercise for money in order that they may win our confidence and dispatch us all the more easily. They also commonly call us barbarians, and stigmatize us more foully than other peoples, by giving us the appellation of Opici. I forbid you to have anything to do with physicians."

In spite of Pliny's claim that for more than six hundred years the Romans had no physicians, there is evidence of medical practitioners from the earliest times. A law dating from the year 433, the *Lex Amela*, prescribed punishment for practitioners who failed to care for sick slaves. Caesar granted citizenship to physicians as part of the reform of A.D. 47. However, it was not until the reign of Septimus Severus (193–211) that laws were passed giving a strict legal basis for the practice of medicine. A system of granting licenses was introduced, and the medical practitioner was made answerable to the state. Abortion and other criminal acts were punished by fines and revocation of licenses. However, during imperial times there was a wide variety of practitioners. Almost anyone could be a "medicus," with little requirement other than reputation. The official physician was called *Archiaturs*, from the Greek meaning "chief healer." By the third century A.D., most of the larger cities in the empire had what were called people's healers.

Although Asclepiades (about 100 B.C.) of Bithynia is regarded as the first Hellenistic physician to influence Roman medical practice, he is overshadowed by two names associated with Rome, the encyclopedist Aurelius Cornelius Celsus (25 B.C.–A.D. 50), upon whose work

De Re Medica historians still rely for the history of early medicine, and the celebrated Claudius Galenus, the last great figure in the medicine of antiquity. Celsus is typical of the educated person of the late Republican period who considered the study of medicine as part of a liberal education. As in the Renaissance, the physician was often also a man of letters. The *De Re Medica,* which was used as a text for medical students until the late nineteenth century, is a virtual encyclopedia of Hellenistic medicine. The work is divided into eight general divisions. The first two deal with diet and the general principles of therapeutics and pathology, the third and fourth internal medicine, the fifth and sixth external diseases, and the final two sections are devoted to surgery.

In the two sections on surgery, Celsus describes the surgical instruments of his time—the scalpel, cup, sound, hook, forceps, speculum, trepan, amputation saw, and spatula. The surgical section includes a complete anatomical account of the human skeleton, with excellent descriptions of the humerus, radius, ulna, tibia, fibula, and tarsus. Celsus recommends that the ideal surgeon be young, of steady hand, accurate eyesight, and unmoved by screams and cries.

Diseases of the eye were widespread in the Roman world and were for the most part treated by "oculari," who were little more than quacks.

In ancient times, there were four ways to treat cataracts. They could be removed completely. The lens could be broken up and left to be absorbed, or the lens could be broken and at once removed by suction. In the following description, Celsus describes the fourth method, that of couching (reclinatiolentis), an operation also known to the Hindus and Egyptians.

If, as the result of a disease or a blow, a humour forms underneath the two tunics in an empty space, it gradually hardens and is an obstacle to the visual power within. There are several species of this lesion; some are curable and some cannot be treated. There is hope if the cataract is small and immobile and if it is the color of sea water or glistening steel and if it is somewhat sensitive to a flash of light. If it is large and if the black part of the eye has lost its natural shape, and if it is sky blue or gold colored and shakes and moves about, then it can seldom ever be cured. The case is worse when the cataract is the result of a severe disease, from severe pains in the head or from a blow of a violent nature. A patient who is advanced in age is not suitable for treatment, as the vision is naturally dulled in addition to the lesion. It is not advisable to treat a child; rather, it is advisable to treat the patient when he is of an intermediate age. Neither a small nor a sunken eye can be satisfactorily treated. And in the cataract itself, there is a certain development. Therefore, one must wait until it is no longer fluid, but appears to have coalesced to some sort of hardness. Before being treated the patient should eat in moderation and drink water for three days beforehand. On the day before treatment, he should abstain from everything. While being treated, the patient should sit opposite the surgeon in a light room, facing the light, and the surgeon should sit on a slightly higher seat; the assistant stands behind and holds the head so that the patient cannot move: for vision can be destroyed permanently by a slight movement. In order to hold the eye as still as possible, wool is put over the opposite eye and bandaged on. The left eye should be operated upon with the left hand. A needle, pointed enough to penetrate without being too fine, should be inserted straight through the two outer tunics at a spot intermediate between the pupil of the eye and the angle adjacent to the temple, away from the middle of the cataract in such a way as to avoid wounding the vein. The needle should not, however, be entered timidly, for it passes into an empty space; and when this is reached even a man of moderate experience cannot be mistaken, for there is then no resistance to pressure. When the spot is reached, the needle is to be sloped against the suffusion itself and should gently rotate there and little by little guide it below the region of the pupil; when the cataract has passed below the pupil it is pressed upon more firmly in order that it may settle below. If it sticks there, the operation has been a success; if it returns to some extent, it should be cut up with the same needle and separated into several pieces, which can then be stowed away more easily singly, and form smaller obstacles to vision. After this the needle should be drawn out straight. Soft wool soaked in egg white should be put on the eye, and above this should be placed something to check inflammation, and bandages above that. The patient must have rest, abstinence, and inunction with soothing medicaments. The day after, he may have food, but it should be liquid in order to avoid the use of the jaws. (De Re Medica, Lib. VI)

Claudius Galenus (130–201), commonly known as Galen, is generally regarded as the most authoritative medical author of the imperial era. His theories and doctrines were never seriously challenged until the seventeenth century. He was born in Pergamos in Asia Minor, which boasted a large temple dedicated to the god of medicine, Aesculapius, and a magnificent library. Galen turned in early life to the study of philosophy and was well grounded in the doctrines of Aristotle and Plato as well as the Stoics and Epicureans. Their influence, especially that of Aristotle, is reflected in his medical writing. After studying medicine in Alexandria, he returned to his birthplace in 157 and became official surgeon to wounded gladiators. The practical experience of treating wounds and fractures was of incalculable worth for his later practice at Rome, where he moved to in 161. For most of the remainder of his life, he acted as court physician for the emperors Marcus Aurelius and Septimus Severus.

During his lifetime, Galen, according to his own account, wrote one hundred twenty-five books on philosophy, mathematics, grammar, and law; unfortunately many of his medical works have been lost. One of his most important works, *The Uses of the Parts of the Body of Man*, was widely used as a basic work for anatomy until the sixteenth century. During the Middle Ages, dissection had been abandoned because it was believed that Galen had written the last word on the subject. Although he advised his students to study human skeletal remains, he believed that human anatomy could be learned from the study of animals, and many of his errors were based upon this false assumption. However, he did dispel the ancient belief that the heart was the origin of the nerves and that the brain was the source of the blood vessels. By cutting the nerves, he obtained the arrest of respiration. He was the first to demonstrate that urine is produced in the kidneys rather than in the bladder as had been previously believed.

His best surviving work, *De Locis Affectis (On the Parts Affected by Disease)*, systematically considers the various organs of the body and the symptoms of the diseases that affect them. He describes disease as "an abnormal affection of the body giving rise to a morbid change in function." Galen classifies diseases by three causes; remote, antecedent or predisposing, and conjunctive or synectic. The first included external causes, such as injuries and abnormalities resulting from air, food, drink, rest, exercise, sleep, excretions, and retentions. The other two causes were internal, the second due to a morbid condition of the body and the third coinciding with the disease.

Following Hippocrates, Galen held that all natural objects were made up of four elements—earth, air, fire, and water. There were also four primary but opposite basic qualities: the hot and the cold, the moist and the dry. The humors were four in number—blood, phlegm, yellow bile, and black bile, originating in the heart, brain, liver, and spleen, respectively. The elements were related to the qualities, and these in turn governed the respective humors. A harmonious mixture of the humors was an ideal state of health. Galen's endorsement of the humoral theory no doubt helped it to survive until the eighteenth century.

In addition to perpetuating the humoral theory, Galen is held to be responsible for three other errors that endured until modern times: the doctrine of vitalism, the false notion of blood movement, and the idea that suppuration is essential to the healing of wounds. For Galen, there existed three kinds of spirits: the natural, the vital, and the animal. The first was located in the liver, where it directed generation, growth, and nutrition. The second, the "vital spirit," was found in the heart, where it directed warmth and life to every part of the body through the arteries. The third, "animal spirit," was located in the brain, where it presided over all the faculties communicating the power of motion and sensation to the various parts of the body by way of the nerves. His belief that the blood passes from the right to the left ventricle by means of invisible pores in the interventricular septum held back genuine medical progress until the time of William Harvey. It was not until the nineteenth-century discovery of asepsis by Joseph Lister that the notion of laudable pus (i.e., that every wound produced pus naturally in the process of healing) was abandoned.

In spite of these inadequacies, Galen synthesized all of the best works of previous Greek writers on medicine. In the treatise *The Best Physician Is Also a Philosopher,* he summarized his position on the ideal physician, who must know logic, in order to think; physics, the science of what is; and ethics, the science of how to act. The demands of this profession, he writes, the long labors required in mastering the science and in the actual study of disease in the living person necessitate extraordinary self-control and the ignoring of the life of pleasure. Galen's basic philosophy, that every part of the body had a God-given proper function, endeared him to the scholars of the Middle Ages. In the following selection, he discusses the relation between structure and function in the major thoracic contents:

I have shown that respiration is useful to animals for the sake of the heart, which to some extent requires the substance of the air and besides needs very greatly to be cooled because of its burning heat. Inspiration cools it by supplying an abundance of the cold quality, expiration by pouring forth the burning hot and, as it were, inflamed and fuliginous material contained in the heart. It is for this reason, too, that the heart has a double motion made up of opposing members, for it attracts during diastole and is emptied during systole. Here you should first observe the foresight of Nature; for since it was better for us to have voices and air is necessary for the production of the voice, she used the otherwise useless and unprofitable expired air as the material for the voice. In my commentaries *On the Voice* I have written a complete account of the instruments of the voice and what sort of motion they have, and as my discourse proceeds, I shall take from that book whatever is necessary for present purposes.

Here Nature first deserves to be praised because she has not caused the heart to attract the outer air directly through the pharynx, but has placed between them the lung as a reservoir for the breath, capable of serving both actions at once. For if the heart in diastole attracted the air from the pharynx and in systole sent the air back into it, the rhythm of respiration and the beat of the heart would have to be the same, and if it were, the animal would encounter many serious difficulties not only in living a good life but in maintaining life itself. The inability to speak very much at a time which would result from such an arrangement would be a considerable hindrance to living a good life, and so would the impossibility of entering the water without fear of suffocation. But the inability to hold the breath while running through smoke, a cloud of dust, or noxious, poisonous air infected by decayed animal matter or from some other cause would quickly threaten life itself and destroy the animal completely. Since, however, the heart does not attract air from the pharynx or directly from outside the body but from the lung, into which it is expelled again, it becomes possible for us frequently to use our voices continuously and frequently to go without breathing with no inconvenience whatever to the heart. If the heart attracted the outer air directly through the pharynx and discharged it directly to the outside again, either one of two evils would necessarily befall us: either we should breathe in noxious air when we ought not, or if we did not breathe in at all, we should be instantly suffocated. These are the reasons, then, why Nature did not make the heart as the only instrument of respiration but surrounded it with the lung and thorax, which were to furnish air to the heart and at the same time produce a voice for the animal. The lung serves besides as, so to speak, a soft jumping ground for the heart, as Plato says, and the thorax as a sort of well-fenced barrier to protect not only the heart but the lung as well.

Nature established the heart in the very center of the cavity of the thorax because she found this place to be most suitable for protection and for uniform refrigeration from the whole body of the lung. It is the common opinion that the heart is not situated exactly in the center but more to the left, but people are deceived by the pulsation apparent in the left breast, where that ventricle lies which is the source of all the arteries. On the right side of the heart, however, there is another ventricle, turned toward the vena cava and the liver, and hence the heart should be said not to lie wholly on the left, but to be placed accurately in the middle, not only in respect to the distance from side to side but also in respect to the other two dimensions of the thorax, depth and length. For the vertebrae behind and the sternum in front are equally distant from the heart, and so are the clavicles above and the diaphragm below. Since, therefore, the heart lies at the mid-point of all the dimensions of the thorax, it attracts equally from all parts of the lung, and since it is very far removed from everything that might reach it from the outside through the thorax, it occupies a very safe position.

The entire middle portion of the thorax is separated off and partitioned by strong (mediastinal) membranes extending longitudinally from above downward. In the rear they are inserted firmly into the vertebrae of the spine and in front into the bone at the middle of the breast (the sternum), which at its lower end has the cartilage called xiphoid near the orifice of the stomach and at its upper end (manubrium) furnishes the attachment for the clavicles. The first and most important use of the membranes is to divide the thorax into two cavities in order that even if one side is badly wounded, as I have told in my book *On the Motion of the Thorax and Lung,* and the work of respiration is thus destroyed on that side, the other cavity, being unharmed, may preserve at least one half of the action. Hence an animal whose thorax is pierced by serious wounds on one side straightway loses half of its voice and respiration, but if both cavities are affected, it will be entirely voiceless and deprived of respiration. (*De Usu Partium,* Lib. VII)

One of the great legacies from Rome to the Western world was its excellent system of public hygiene and its hospitals. The city of Rome was provided with fresh water by the fourteen great aqueducts, ten of which were built before A.D. 110, supplying the city with 40 million gallons of drinking water daily. Most private homes had main service pipes equipped with cisterns and taps. As described by the Roman writer and engineer Frontonius, who was educated in Alexandria, the Roman system of aqueducts in the first century was not surpassed until the nineteenth century. Public baths and fountains as well as sewers were found in all of the major cities of the empire. City officials were commissioned to ensure the purity of the water, and the lead piping was under constant surveillance. Settling tanks and other purification methods were used on a large scale. Although it was suspected at that time that lead pipes were not the best conduits of water, it was not until the eighteenth century that British physician Sir

George Boher alerted the public to the dangers of lead poisoning from this source.

The Baths of Caracalla could accommodate sixteen hundred patrons; those of Diocletian contained three thousand rooms.

The Cloaca Maxima in Rome, which is used to this day, carried both sewage and surface water to the Tiber. The Cloaca was actually a vaulted canal capable of being navigated. Roman ruins in Timgad in North Africa display well-ordered hygienic and sanitary systems. This small city boasted fifteen public baths as well as ornately decorated public toilets and latrines. One such public lavatory contained some twenty-six stone-covered seats, each enclosed by stone dolphins and constantly drained by a fountain in the center.

The construction and administration of hospitals were also a part of the Roman medical world, although many were used for slaves and in military installations. Ruins excavated in Germany and Austria show well-designed buildings capable of accommodating forty sick wards constructed as long corridors surrounding a dining room, medical staff kitchens, and apothecary shops.

One of the problems that has perplexed historians since the time of Augustine has been the decline of the Roman Empire. Not a few of the theories are related to medicine. The failure of the Romans to perfect their drainage system in the environs of the city and the resultant enervating malaria has been cited. The use of lead pipes and leaden containers for wine is offered as another explanation: the populace was gradually poisoned. A number of theories involve genetics. Early in this century, American historian Tenney Frank concluded that the influx of Greek and Oriental slaves eventually changed the entire character of the Romans, causing them to lose identity and national pride. Another theory suggests that the Romans ought to have dominated the barbarians by intermarrying with them.

Yet long before the death of the last emperor in the West in 476 (he was killed by the Germanic chieftan Odovacer), Roman medicine had been in a state of decline. The severe measures against the use of magic for curative purposes by the emperors of the third century are indicative of the deterioration of medicine. Even during the first century, when the practice of medicine reached a certain perfection, there were those who did not hesitate to criticize it. The Spanish-born epigrammatist Marcus Martialis wrote of the practitioners of his day:

Dialus was once a physician,
But later became a mortician:
Bed rest, as before,
He prescribes, only more—
An exceedingly minor transition.
Occulist once and now a gladiator
No change, except the new arena's greater.

(Tr. Ker.)

4

The Middle Ages

MEDIEVAL OR Middle Ages generally connotes an era of civilization in decline; a dark chapter in the history of mankind. Yet as an eminent historian once remarked, these ages were never so dark as our ignorance of them. Historically, the arbitrary division of the past into ancient, medieval, and modern is the result of two movements that mark the end of the Middle Ages: the Renaissance and the Reformation. For the humanists of the Renaissance, the preceding age was one of obscurity and darkness because it lacked the classical heritage of Greece and Rome. For the Protestant theologians of the sixteenth century, it was a benighted period because the light of the Gospel had been obscured by the pretentions of the papacy. It was not, however, until the seventeenth century that this historical period became understood.

Since that time, it has been customary to use the term "Middle Ages" to designate the political, national, and cultural life in the West that began with the appearance of two new peoples, long confined to the frontiers of the Roman Empire: the Germanic tribes to the North and the Arabs to the South. The Germanic peoples established a number of kingdoms on the ruins of the Roman Empire: the Vandals in North Africa, the Goths in Spain and Italy, the Franks in Gaul and Germany, and the Angles and Saxons in Britain. In addition to common tribal practices, an emphasis on kinship and the practice of annual assemblies to settle legal matters, the new people of the West came to share a common religious belief, and it was Christianity, more than any other factor, that gave them a sense of community.

This sharing of common religious faith was equally apparent among

54

the peoples who invaded the empire from the south: the Arabs. Although often regarded as a religion enforced by the sword, Islam was in essence extremely attractive. Its simplicity, especially when contrasted with Judaism and Christianity, to which it was closely related, was one of the chief reasons for its rapid spread. It was the basic belief of all Muhammadans that there was one God, Allah, and that Muhammad was his prophet. Allah was the creator of all things, visible and invisible. He was both just and merciful, and would in the hereafter punish the evil and reward the good. Allah demanded a high moral code that was universal and similar to the Decalogue. Concern for the poor, orphans, and widows was obligatory. Once a year, the month of Ramadan was a period of fasting and abstinence. There were certain dietary regulations; no pork was allowed, and the consumption of wine or other intoxicating liquor was proscribed.

Muhammad had little to say concerning medicine. As an earlier biographer said, "his mission was to make known to us the prescriptions of the divine law and not to instruct us in medicine and the common practices of ordinary life." Early Muslim writings on medicine actually deal with such matters as visiting the sick and providing them with spiritual consolations, amulets, talismans, and magic formulas. It was not until the Arabs came into contact with the Hellenistic world that anything resembling scientific medicine is found.

The Arabs, united through doctrines of Islam, eventually conquered what remained of the Roman Empire in Africa and the Middle East. Muslim rule was established over the greater part of Spain as well as Sicily. By the ninth century, what had been the Roman Empire was divided into three distinct political and cultural blocks: Byzantium, Islam, and Latin Christendom. It was the interrelationship between these areas that determined much of what is called the Middle Ages. This interrelationship is especially evident in the realm of medicine. It is to these three cultures that we must turn to understand the medieval world.

Greatly reduced by the loss of its provinces in the West and the territories now in Muslim hands, the Byzantine Empire struggled to maintain its political and cultural heritage. The emperor was looked on as an agent of God. Although the state provided a highly developed educational system based on the study of classical literature, it tended to be imitative rather than creative. This was especially true in medicine.

Oreibsios (326–403) is the most well known of the Byzantine physicians. The personal physician to Emperor Julian the Apostate, he compiled an encyclopedia that contained many of the works of Galen and other Hellenistic authors. Of the seventy volumes included in this massive work, more than a third are extant. Oreibsios was strongly opposed to superstition, which was prevalent, and wrote a number of tracts against magicians, charmers, and fabricators of amulets. The fourth century saw an incredible increase in the use of magical charms and amulets to combat disease and sickness. Emperor Julian, who attempted to destroy Christianity by replacing Christ with the god of healing, was deeply influenced by the magical arts.

Aetios of Amida (502–575), who is regarded as one of the first Christian physicians of note, is also an example of how strong was the belief in magic in spite of Christianity. It must be recalled that even Galen was not above advising the use of amulets as medical cures, recommending them for headaches, overindulgence, and fevers. Pagan deities were replaced by Christian saints. Aetios urged that in preparing a plaster one should intone the following prayer: "The God of Abraham, the God of Isaac, the God of Jacob give power to this medicament." St. Blase is called upon to remove obstructions from the throat "As Jesus Christ drew Lazarus from the sepulchre and Jonah out of the whale, so Blase, martyr and servant of Christ, commands either come up or down."

By the seventh century, a whole litany of saints, each with a special curative attribute, had evolved in the Eastern Empire. The twins Cosmos and Damien, who had suffered martyrdom in Sicily in the third century, were the most popular of the medical saints.

In spite of his use of charms and incantations, Aetios remained within the rational school of Alexandrian medicine. His work on ophthalmology, in which he describes some sixty-one diseases of the eye, is considered the most comprehensive in antiquity. In his writing are found the earliest references to the use of camphor, cloves, and other eastern drugs.

Alexander of Tralles (525–605) is regarded as the most celebrated physician of Byzantium. Benefiting from the temporary resurgence of the empire under Justinian, who for a time succeeded in governing the West, Alexander traveled extensively in the reconquered territories of Africa, Italy, Spain, and Gaul. He eventually settled in Rome and wrote a considerable body of medical literature. Much of it was translated from the original Greek into Latin, Syrian, Hebrew, and Arabic. His most important work, *Twelve Books of Medicine,* exerted a great influence throughout the Middle Ages. It was highly regarded at the school of Salerno. Although an eclectic, Alexander was largely influenced by the writings of Galen, especially in his support of the humoral theory.

A third important figure in the Byzantine world of medicine is Paul of Aegina (625–690). He is regarded as the last of the great Greek physicians. His lifetime spanned the years of the greatest expansion of Islam into Byzantine territory. In 636, a powerful Muslim army defeated Greek forces at the battle of Yarmuk, a reversal that marked an accelerated breakup of much of the empire. In 641, Arab forces captured Mosul in the Tigris; five years later, Alexandria fell; by 649, the followers of Muhammad had secured the island of Cyprus. Paul remained in Alexandria even after the Arab conquest. His greatest work was a seven-volume encyclopedia of medicine. The sixth volume of the work was devoted to surgery and exercised considerable influence in both the Arab world and the West, where it was a prescribed text at the University of Paris. The work displayed a wide knowledge of surgical practice describing tracheotomy, excision of tonsils and nasal polyps, resection of the ribs in emphysema, and catheterization. His work on obstetrics was looked upon as authoritative during much of the Middle Ages; yet his failure to describe sufficiently cephalic and podalic version is regarded by some to have been responsible for the disappearance of this type of delivery during the medieval period.

The absorption of almost one-third of the Roman Empire by the Arabs created a unique culture that survives to this day. After 750, the vast area conquered by the successors of Muhammad was ruled from two centers: Baghdad in the East and Cordova in the West. By the ninth century, Baghdad had a population of eight hundred thousand and was regarded as the political, cultural, and intellectual center of the Muslim world. Cordova, with a population of one-half million, boasted the largest library in Europe. Both cities were centers of an astonishing intellectual activity. By insisting that the Koran be learned only in Arabic, the conquest produced a common language that reached from Spain to India. Practically all the worlds' cultural traditions were united: Hellenistic, Mesopotamian, Egyptian, and Indian. The accumulated knowledge provided the Arabs with a collection of scientific knowledge unsurpassed anywhere until modern times. By the ninth century, Arabic had become an international language of science. After assimilating the best of Hellenistic traditions preserved in Persia and Byzantium, Arabian scholars added a new rich dimension by borrowing from India and the Far East. The use of anesthetics by way of inhalation, animal gut for closing wounds, and clinical instruction in hospitals are but a few of the advances made by the Arabs.

Historians trace the origins of Arabian medicine to the Persian school of Jundishapur, capital of the Sassanians. Staffed largely by Nestorian Christians driven from the Byzantine Empire, the school was characterized by a mingling of Hellenistic and Indian learning, much of it translated into Syriac. In addition to the works of Hippocrates and Galen, the texts of Rufus of Ephesus, Oribasius, Paul of Aegiria, and Alexander of Tralles were highly regarded. The Nestorian Christian Hunian ibn Ishaq (809–877) translated the basic works into Arabic and thus formed the foundation of the later Muslim Canon of medical literature.

Two Persian Muslims, Rhazes, or Al Razi (860–932), and Avicenna (980–1036), dominate the medical world of the Eastern Caliphate. Rhazes was born in the village of Ray, a few miles from modern Teheran. A musician, he did not turn to medicine until his later years. He was a practitioner as well as a theorist and authored more than a hundred tracts on practical medicine, many written when he was chief physician at the newly founded hospital in Baghdad. His description of smallpox and measles, introduced into the West under the title *De Pestilentia,* was for centuries a standard work, as was his monograph on kidney stones. His most well-known work, the *Hawi,* or, as Latinized, the *Continens Rhazes,* was compiled after his death by his students, and is his longest and most important work. The book, which was first printed in Brescia in 1486, is a compendium of various tracts, original clinical histories, and experiments in therapeutics. Rhazes is credited with having introduced the use of mercurial ointment into the Arabian and Western worlds.

The greatest name in this golden age of Arabian culture was undoubtedly that of Ibn Sina, or Avicenna, philosopher, physician, poet, and diplomat. He was born near Bokhara of parents who were members of the Ismaili sect. A precocious child, he soon mastered the Arabian classics, geometry, jurisprudence, and logic. On his own, he soon surpassed his instructors and studied theology, physics, mathematics, and medicine. At the age of sixteen, he was practicing as a doctor, and by eighteen, his reputation was such that he was summoned to the court of the ruler of Sainani (Samini). Subsequently, he moved to enter the service of the ruler of Khiva, one of several sultans he was to serve as vizier. His chief philosophical work is entitled *As-Sifa,* or, in Latin, *Sufficientiae.* It had a profound influence on the medieval scholars Roger Bacon, Thomas Aquinas, and Albert the Great, among others. Many of his works on medicine were actually written in verse. The *Qanun,* or *Canon of Medicine,* is Avicenna's largest and most famous work. It is divided into five books: general principles, drugs, diseases of various organs, diseases that affect the entire body such as fevers, and compounded medicines. The following describes the various types of pulse:

With regard to the compound pulses, some have distinctive names and some do not. A pulse which is increased in length, breadth and depth is called large. When all of these dimensions are smaller, it is called small. The moderate pulse is the mean between the two.

A pulse which is increased in breadth and depth is called thick; one which is smaller in these two dimensions is called slender. The medium pulse is the mean between the two.

There are three varieties of the quality of impact: strong, which resists the finger during expansion; weak, which has the opposite character; and the intermediate.

There are three varieties with regard to the duration of the cycle: rapid or short or swift, where the movement is completed in a short time; slow or sluggish or long, which is the opposite; and the intermediate, or moderately quick pulse.

There are three varieties with regard to the consistence of the artery: soft or easily compressible; hard, firm or incompressible; and one of moderate compressibility.

The full or high pulse seems to be overfull of humor and gives the impression that it needs liberating. The empty or low pulse is contrary in character. There is an intermediate between the two.

The pulse may feel hot, cold, or intermediate. A hurried or dense pulse is one in which the period between the two successive beats is short; a sluggish pulse, where the period is prolonged. There is a mean between the two. This period of time is distinguished from the contraction-period, but if contraction cannot be perceived it can be estimated from the period of time between the two expansions. In this case, it is reckoned from the times of the two extremes.

The equality or inequality of the pulse is reckoned according to whether or not the two successive pulses are similar or dissimilar, there being a difference of size (large or small), strength (strong or weak), swiftness (rapid or slow, prompt or sluggish), hardness or softness, until it happens that the second expansion of the first pulse is overtaken by the first of the next (due to excess of innate heat), or is weaker than the next (excess of weakness).

This discourse could be expanded to cover the inequality or equality of the pulse in regard to the three variants in the other features of the pulse afore-mentioned, but it is sufficient to consider them solely with regard to strength.

A regular or equal pulse in the strict sense is one which is regular in all of these respects; if it is regular only in one feature, it is so specified. Thus we speak of a pulse as regular or equal in strength or regular in speed. In the same way, a pulse is irregular either in all respects or only in one.

With regard to orderliness or disorderliness, there are two forms: the pulse may be irregularly orderly or irregularly disorderly. The orderly pulse main-tains orderly succession. This occurs in one of two ways. The orderliness is absolute, where every feature is maintained; or cyclical, where there are two or more irregularities which keep repeating in cycles, as if there were two cycles simultaneously, or superposed, so that the original order reappears.

It is apparent that the tenth feature belongs here and its omission can be justified.

The pulse has a musical character. In the art of music, sounds are jux-taposed in orderly relations of loudness and softness which are repeated at regular intervals; rates of utterance vary—some sounds coming close to one another, and others are far apart; the attack may be abrupt or gentle, sharp or dull. The notes may be sounded clearly or indefinitely; they may be strong or weak; the volume may be full or "thin." The rhythm of the sequence of the sounds may be regular or irregular.

All of the above features are characteristic of the pulse. The intervals between the beats, or the successions, may be harmonious or inharmonious. So, too, the irregularities may be orderly or disorderly. It is orderly when there is a proper relation of strength and weakness. It is disorderly if there is not.

All of this concerns the question of order and regularity.

Indeed, Galen discussed the metre of the pulse, or its rhythm along the lines of musical nomenclature. Thus, we would have double time, three-four time, common time, four-five time, five-six time, and so on. For those who have a sensitive touch and a keen sense of rhythm, with musical training, such observations could be correlated in the mind. I am surprised to think how many of such relations could be perceived by the sense of touch, and yet I am confident that it can be done if one is habituated to the use of it, and can apportion metre and beats of time. On the other hand, since these variations all belong to inequality and disorderliness, it is not necessary to define them particularly.

Even if the preceding details cannot be perceived, at least the relation between period of expansion and period of pause can be appreciated, as well as the relation between the total duration of beat and the total duration of pause. Under this heading, then, we place: first total period of pulse; next total period; period of expansion; period of pause; period of expansion plus period of pause; period of contraction plus period of pause; period of expansion; period of contraction. A relation of period of expansion; period of contraction; or, period of first pause; period of second pause, is not important.

Metre (rhythm, beat, or accent) is good (eurhythm) or bad (arhythm) according to the musical analogy. There are three kinds of arhythm. The first is pararhythm, where the beat is altered only slightly and temporarily, for example, where an adult has a metre which is only natural in youth or where a child has a rhythm which is proper for an adult. The second type is heterorhythm, where the change is greater in degree; for example, where a youth had the metre of an old man. The third type is etrhythm. The change in this case is altogether different; the metre does not conform to the human type at all. A great change in metre denotes a great change in the bodily state. (*Canon*, Lib. I, Pars II, Thesis 3)

In the Western Caliphate, two figures stand out above all others in the field of medicine. Ibn Ruschd (1126–98), better known through his Latinized name Averroës, and his student the Jewish Moses Maimonides (1135–1204). Both were natives of Cordova and eminent philosophers as well as physicians. Averroës, the son of a judge, distinguished himself as a student in theology, jurisprudence, mathematics, and philosophy as well as medicine. He was appointed physician to the caliph in 1182. His fame as a philosopher rests upon his attempt to explain the doctrines of Islam in terms of the metaphysics of Aristotle. He believed that Aristotle was the completer of human learning and the author of a system of supreme truth. His efforts to reconcile the revelations of the Koran with the pagan philosopher led to his being accused of heresy, and he was forced to flee to Marrakesh in Morocco, where he died in 1198. The Latin scholars referred to him as "the commentator," and his ideas had a profound influence upon Aquinas and other Christian scholars. In the *Divine Comedy*, Dante places Averroës in Limbo while relegating Muhammad to Hell. Aristotelian ideas dominate his medical system, which is summarized in his *General Rules of Medicine,* known in the West as the *Colliget.*

The most famous Jewish scholar of the medieval period is Moses Maimonides (Rabbi Moses ben Maimon). Like his teacher, Averroës, he attempted to reconcile his religion with the newly rediscovered writings of Aristotle, to bridge the gap between Talmudic knowledge and Hellenic science. To this end, he published a number of works, or commentaries. In 1168, there appeared his *Commentary on the Mishnah,* an interpretation of Jewish law and theology that is used to this day. His most well known theological work is the *Guide for the Perplexed,* a series of instructional letters on the nature of God, the existence of God, the problem of evil, and the communication between God and man. The work is a synthesis of Greek, Arabian, and Jewish thought.

Maimonides was forced to flee Spain because of the intolerance of the fanatic Almohades, who captured Cordova in 1148. After a period of time in Morocco, he settled in Egypt, where, in 1185, he was appointed personal physician to the Great Saladin. Maimonides' most well known medical work is a collection of aphorisms from Galen entitled *Aphorismen Moses.* Some five later editions of the work were printed in Europe between 1498 and 1579. In the following section, Maimonides establishes the rules for phlebotomy, or bloodletting:

The following three criteria are needed to determine the necessity for phlebotomy: first, the severity of the illness at present or that which is ready to develop, second, the patient should be neither too young nor too old, third, his resistence should be sufficiently strong.

If the patient's arteries are broad and large, and if his body is somewhat lean and he is not too pale and his flesh is not too moist, then he may be phlebotomized without fear or danger. For someone with the opposite conditions, he should be phlebotomized only with the utmost care and precaution.

A youth under 14 or a man over the age of 70 should not be phlebotomized. In addition, the facial appearance should be taken into account. Many people who are only 60 years old cannot tolerate phlebotomy at all whereas others who are 70 can tolerate it well because they are strong and have a plentiful supply of blood.

If someone wishes to phlebotomize a patient in the springtime, he should be closely examined and questioned. If any of his organs are weak, then the filling with blood will tend to be toward the side of the body in which the weak organ is situated. In this case, the patient is phlebotomized from the side from which the organ is attracting fluids. If none of his organs are weak, he may be phlebotomized from either side.

The conditions which prohibit bloodletting, despite an adequate supply of blood are: spasms, severe insomnia, anginal type pain, marked warmth either in the very warm areas or in the very cold ones, or a noticeably warm and dry constitution, soft and flabby flesh, flesh with openings that are patent where rapid dissolution occurs, extreme obesity, inordinate anxiety, fear in a youngster or an elderly person, stomach pains, nausea, bad liquids which irritate, diarrhea or colitis. If a patient is noticeably filled with blood together with one of the previously mentioned conditions and cannot progress in healing without bloodletting, then he should be phlebotomized with great caution and care. Only a few of the prohibitive symptoms are mentioned here. They all, however, tend to weaken the strength of the patient.

It is doubtful that phlebotomy is ever advisable if the body is full of unmetabolized liquids. In such a case, bloodletting is dangerous because the patient's strength will diminish and weaken to the point that it will be impossible to restore the body to its previous health especially if a fever is present.

If a person has good blood but not enough of it, and if raw liquids are in abundance, one should not do anything which might exhaust him. He should not be purged or placed in a steambath. The reason for this is that phlebotomy would remove the healthy blood and draw out the infected blood gathered in the main arteries of the liver and divert it into the entire system.

In addition, a purgative medication given to a patient in this condition will produce intestinal pain, irritation and collapse. Therefore one cannot empty something just because it is present in a certain amount. Liquids will close and obstruct passageways because they are viscous. For this reason, the patient should not exercise or take a steambath. It is appropriate to thin his viscous liquids and to dissolve them with remedies that will not produce too much warmth.

An otherwise healthy person in whom there are signs of an abundance of body liquids should not be bled under any circumstances. In such a person, the withholding of food alone may be adequate. After this treatment diminishing the alimentary intake alone may suffice, and following this the softening of the stool may be adequate, or purgation, or numerous steambaths, or physical exercise alone, or much massage, according to the tolerance and custom of the individual. Any of these may obviate the need for bloodletting.

With regard to phlebotomy, it is necessary to be familiar with the subject and recognize an individual with little blood. In this case, he should first be treated until his liquids have become replenished. After the liquids have been replenished, the vessel may be lanced and the patient fed following the phlebotomy. A second phlebotomy may be performed if the patient requires it. This method of therapy is most advantageous in people whose blood is turbid or contains raw, viscous sediments.

If it should happen that a phlebotomy patient's artery bursts or menstruation or diarrhea sets in, the phlebotomy should be discontinued. If the amount already removed is sufficient, then nature can be relied upon to complete the entire process. If it is insufficient then the patient is phlebotomized again to withdraw an amount twice as great as that usually required.

If phlebotomy is necessary but a stomach ailment sets in, it should be postponed until the food producing the upset is digested and its wastes are excreted from the body. If diarrhea or vomiting occurs, the postponement of the phlebotomy is absolutely essential.

If the superfluous chyme particles are evenly distributed throughout the body organs, all should be emptied. The most reliable method is phlebotomy and, after it are the other types of beneficial emptying such as blood losses through menstruation or hemorrhage. In addition to this, the patient should be exercised, massaged, steambathed and his diet supervised.

If an excess of blood exists in the body, it is wise to eliminate it rapidly before it pours itself into one or more of the major organs. It is therefore not correct to withhold venesection when the need arises by day or night.

Sometimes the blood suddenly hemorrhages because of its excess before any organ putrefies and its function ceases completely. In such a case, the patient suffers immense damage which is characteristic of apoplexy. This damage is produced by the sudden and copious flow of blood to the brain. If one observes signs of an abundance of blood together with adequate strength of the three powers, referring to the spiritual, animal and natural powers of the body, phlebotomy should be performed without hesitation.

If the body has an excess of blood which is at the boiling point, then acute fever will develop. In such a case, blood should be quickly removed until fainting occurs, after the patient's tolerance has been established. I personally have removed approximately a "litre" of blood on the second, third or fourth day after the onset of the illness.

It is best, to remove small amounts of blood several times, over one to three days, from a patient who is weak but who requires that some blood be let from him. He should be fed easily digestable foods following the phlebotomy. One should be very cautious not to remove a large amount of blood rapidly without there being a valid reason.

If one intends to perform a normal, unavoidable phlebotomy, the venesection should be done immediately, on the same day. However, if one intends to phlebotomize the side opposite the illness, it is advisable to wait until the second or third day. At all times, the patient's strength should be taken into consideration.

During venesection, while the blood is flowing, the patient should be observed at all times for changes in his countenance, especially if he is suffering from a warm inflammation. The sediment of the shed blood should also be examined after the phlebotomy has ended. It is very important to examine the pulse. If it is changing in its fulness or rhythm, the phlebotomy should be terminated immediately. Venesection should cease immediately if the patient becomes faint.

A moderate quantity of blood should be removed until change occurs in all illnesses. If possible, this should be done on the first or second day and so forth, except if one intends to phlebotomize the patient until he collapses.

If you are dealing with a severe illness and if the patient is strong enough, then anyone who has practiced and studied the art of medicine should not withhold bloodletting. He should not avoid this type of therapy even if the signs of the filling of the body with blood are lacking but rather be guided only by the strength and severity of the illness. The same applies for purgation of the bowels or induction of emesis where one considers either the excess of bad liquids other than blood, or one is guided by the strength and severity of the illness because it is diverted to the opposite side thus supporting the patient's strength.

Bloodletting always requires the renewal of strength sufficient to replace the amount of blood that was removed. Reduction of strength is, second to phlebotomy, the most dangerous part of this procedure. In high fevers that occur due to deficient dissolution of bad liquids, phlebotomy is safe and is far from being dangerous because in most cases the strength of the patient is adequate. In other illnesses, however, phlebotomy is dangerous and a patient can be harmed.

Venesection is a necessity at the very beginning of the following illnesses: podagra, arthritis, cephalagia, melancholia, repetitive hemoptysis or a tendency to suffer from this illness, frequent choking, pneumonia, convulsions, hepatitis or severe ophthalmia. The same applies to those whose hemorrhoidal bleeding has ceased. In this case, phlebotomy can be performed with relative ease and peace of mind. A woman whose menstrual periods have stopped or someone who often develops epistaxis should be rapidly phlebotomized after strength and age are considered.

It is appropriate to remove blood from a patient with inflammatory tiredness until he becomes faint if there is no contraindication. One should then examine to see if there is a stretching or sticking pain in the breast, in the spine, or in the small backbone. In such cases the basilic vein should be bled. If the patient feels pain in the head or neck, blood should be taken from the "folded vein" which is the cephalic vein. If he senses the tiredness equally throughout the entire body, then the median antecubital vein should be bled.

If a nerve tears in its width, then the patient is in danger of contracture if an infection also develops. Therefore, the patient should be bled without restraint and more blood should be removed than is usually removed for another illness. He should have the most easily tolerated diet possible and should remain calm. In addition, warm oil should be rubbed from the site of the wound to the roots of the nerve in question, up to the back and up to the neck.

One who phlebotomizes should bleed the patient during the descent of the fever, day and night. He should be extremely careful in taking blood while food is still in the stomach and/or major arteries, which have not yet completed digestion. On the other hand, in the patient who has no fever, as in the case of ophthalmia, the best time for phlebotomy is at the moment of greatest pain. If there is no pain, then the best time is in the middle of the day one hour after awakening.

One should not deliberate much concerning the number of days that have passed since the beginning of an illness in a person who requires a phlebotomy, because of this illness, as to whether it is the fourth or fifth day. If the patient is in need of bloodletting it should be done at once, even if it is only the second day since the outset of the illness. As in all cases, one should consider the severity of the illness, the overall strength of resistance of the patient, the age of the patient and the time.

In all illness of the subclavicular region, it is advantageous to phlebotomize the basilic vein. The best site for phlebotomy in the case of illness of the supraclavicular region is the axillary vein.

For illnesses of organs above the liver, one should venesect from the antecubital vein. For illnesses of organs below the liver, one should bleed from the popliteal vein and from the saphenous vein.

Inflammations of the side, the lung or diaphragm, or spleen, liver or stomach are all clearly benefited by bloodletting from the basilic vein. For inflammations of organs below the aforementioned ones such as the adnexal organs for the loins, the urinary bladder and the uterus, it is healthy to phlebotomize from the knee and above the ankle. The kidneys are considered as if they are in between these two groups of organs. Therefore such patients benefit from phlebotomy from the antecubital vein because of its closeness to the site of the inflammation as well as if the whole body is filled with blood. However, if the inflammation in the kidneys becomes prolonged and chronic, then one should phlebotomize the vein within the knee or near the ankle.

If there is pain in the ischial area resulting from an excess of blood, then therapy should not be started until it is eliminated. It is not sufficient to remove blood only from the leg without letting blood from the elbow region.

Bloodletting from the saphenous vein or from one within the knee will cure sciatica on the same day that one removes the blood from the leg, especially if the illness developed secondary to overfilling with blood. In such a case suction cups are of no use at all.

If one wishes to drain blood which flows from openings in arteries related to hemorrhoids, then the leg veins should be phlebotomized. If one desires to stimulate menstrual blood one should also phlebotomize these veins. If a vessel in the uterus bursts, however, from corrosion or overfilling and if the woman is hemorrhaging and one wishes to stop it, one should phlebotomize the veins in the arms because this is not menstrual blood.

At the beginning of an inflammation of the liver, chest or lung, one should phlebotomize the basilic vein of the right arm. If it cannot be located, one should use the cephalic vein. As a final resort one should phlebotomize the jugular vein under the tongue.

If the illness is in the neck, one should let blood from the arm or forehead. For infections of the kidneys or uterus, one should phlebotomize the vessel in the venous plexus of the knee. If this is not possible, then one should use the vessel around the ankle and this is the saphenous. For illnesses of the spleen, one should phlebotomize the left arm. (*Aphorismi Raby Moysis,* XII, *Plebotomia*)

In the West, where the decline of Roman civilization was much more in evidence than in the East, the loss of the Greek language greatly affected the knowledge and practice of medicine. After the sixth century, medical practice was, to a great extent, limited to the monasteries. There are some isolated references to the legal status of the practitioners as established under Roman rule, but they indicate the near extinction of licensed medicine. Visigothic law in Italy included provisions for the protection of patients against incompetent physicians. The monk Cassiodorus, who, before he retired to a monastery in 540, was an official at the court of Theodoric, created a library that included many of the medical works of antiquity. Cassiodorus made it a rule that the monks in his foundation familiarize themselves with Dioscorides and the Latin versions of Hippocrates and Galen. His efforts to form a center for learning in Rome, a university modeled after those of Alexandria and Nisibis, in Syria, came to nought largely because of the political instability of the times. As a matter of fact, it was Cassiodorus who first introduced the monastic practice of translating and copying the classical texts of Greece and Rome. The monastic *scriptoria* made possible the eventual recovery of the knowledge of the classical world, thus laying the foundations for scholarship and institutionalized learning. In the ninth century, the famed monastery of Monte Cassino possessed the nucleus of a medical library, and the monastic schools of this period record the practice of instruction in elementary medicine. The Carolingian Renaissance, by reviving the study of classical literature, laid the groundwork for an eventual recovery of the medical knowledge of antiquity. Charles the Great, although he disdained practitioners of his time, nevertheless enacted legislation in 805 that prescribed the teaching of the medical arts for monastic students.

What little literary reference there is to early Germanic medicine indicates that it was largely entrusted to women healers. Although male healers were active, their services usually were called upon only in times of warfare. The lack of a trained corps of medical practitioners during the early Middle Ages explains the severity of local laws against malpractice and the Church's later prohibition of surgery by the clergy.

Hence, for the most part, early medieval medicine was a crude mixture of superstition and folklore. Prior to their conversion to Christianity, the Germanic peoples sought cures through a variety of effigies, talismans, and amulets associated with the Norse gods. Sacred trees and springs possessed curative powers. The *sculptilia pede facta* (carved images of human feet placed at crossroads) were looked upon as restorers of health. The mandragora was especially regarded as a magical drug. It was often soaked in water, wine, or beer to prepare a magical potion and was sprinkled on humans as well as domestic animals. Betony was considered to possess the power to comfort the ears, spleen, eyes, and stomach and cure dropsy, the bite of a mad dog, and ague. It was believed that whoever saw a marigold early in the morning would be free from fever throughout the day. If carried about, mugwort would prevent fever, as would rubbing with plantain. That the hair of the dog was good for its bite is an expression that still survives, especially for those who have imbibed too deeply.

In addition to herbs, minerals and stones were used for their curative powers. Pulverized magnetic stone taken with milk was believed to prevent melancholia. Amagrad worn about the neck on a chain saved the wearer from epilepsy. Onyx fastened to the throat stimulated the salivary glands. Amber was used against cerebral troubles. Sapphire mixed with milk cured ulcers and stopped excessive perspiration.

As in Byzantium, Christianity replaced pagan deities and talismans with relics of venerated saints and ritual exorcism. Disease was often attributed to diabolical possession. In the writings of Constantine of

Africa, a renowned eleventh-century physician, there is a curious reference to sexual impotence resulting from witchcraft. Among suggested means for breaking the spell are sprinkling the house with dog's blood and fumigating the bedroom with the bile of a fish. Almost every disease or malady found its cure through the intercession of this or that particular saint. The twin saints, Cosmos and Damien, third-century martyrs and physicians, enjoyed a widespread cult in both the East and the West. St. Sebastian and St. Roch were invoked in times of plague. St. Blase was called upon for protection against diseases of the throat. A curious relic of the Middle Ages, the so-called royal touch, lasted in England until the time of the Hanoverians. It was believed that a touch from the royal hand had curative powers. An elaborate liturgy carried out in the cathedral on specific feast days, Easter, Christmas, and Pentecost had developed in this regard by the eleventh century.

By about the year 1000, western Europe began to recover from the devastations of the barbarian invasions. The Vikings had settled in Normandy, Sicily, and Kiev; the Magyars were reduced to the area of Hungary. The millenary is often cited as a watershed between the Dark Ages and the awakening of western Europe, for during the next three centuries there developed a civilization that was in many ways unique. It was supranational in that it lacked a political or national focus, and it created for several centuries a homogeneous culture formed by teachers, thinkers, and writers. It is known in history as the Age of the Schoolman. Its great intellectual achievement was a synthesis of Christian, Hellenistic, and Arabian thought dominated by dialecticism and rationalism. In this world, where the study of theology dominated all other disciplines, there was little room for genuine advance in medicine.

The intellectual awakening was preceded by a number of technological advances that explain the shift of population centers from the Mediterranean to northern Europe, for example the discoveries that certain crops (rye and wheat) could be planted and harvested twice a year and that the three-field system greatly increased the production of food. The invention of the horseshoe, stirrup, and horse collar, unknown to the ancient world, increased transportation possibilities. The pulling power of the horse was quadrupled. Water power for milling as well as the invention of the windmill provided energy for the emerging cities. Above all, the discovery of a new type of plow, the mouldboard, made possible the tilling of the heavily overgrown soil of northern Europe. With the invention of the spinning wheel, cheap cloth became available, and the discovery of the button changed clothes. During the late ninth century, a peculiar type of social organization had developed that was known as feudalism. Its appearance was due to the almost complete lack of legal institutions and centralized government. Based upon land tenure, a great deal of economic and military power was in the hands of an heriditary nobility. Many of the social institutions associated with feudalism lasted until the French Revolution.

A disproportionate number of physicians were clergymen. Until the fifteenth century, celibacy was a requirement for medical doctors at many universities. Yet it was this fact that gave the medical practitioner a sense of vocation or calling. The strong religious ethos of the Middle Ages placed upon the physician not only an aura of sanctity; it demanded that he perform certain duties toward his fellowman as a God-given obligation. It has been said that the medical profession has retained to this day this sense of vocation, more than any other profession. The Synod of Tours, in 1163, passed legislation that forbade clergy to perform surgery, *Ecclesia abhorret a sanguine* (the Church recoils from blood). This law was reinforced by later legislation, resulting in a separation between surgeon and physician. Surgeons were for the most part unlettered craftsmen, barbers, blood letters, and, too often, quacks.

The intellectual revival that began in the eleventh century was to lead to our most valuable legacy from the Middle Ages: the university. Nothing like it had existed in the ancient worlds of Greece and Rome, and they were not found in the Far East. Historians are still in dispute about their precise origin. During the eleventh and twelfth centuries, as the older monastic and cathedral schools, which are traceable to the reform of Charles the Great, began to decline, they were replaced by new-school scholars who banded together and drew up constitutions to protect themselves and their students from the encroachments of the local clergy and civic authorities. As an organization, the university resembled the medieval guild, which was already in evidence among the craftsmen, merchants, and physicians. In a sense, it was symptomatic of the deep sense of corporateness that was so much in evidence in Europe during the twelfth and thirteenth centuries. The same organizational trend is also seen in the beginnings of the municipal laws and the rise of cities.

In the Middle Ages, the expression "universitas" had a different meaning from its current one of an institution of higher learning offering a wide choice of studies. It was essentially a corporation or aggregation of students and faculty who were licensed to grant certificates of achievement following a regulated course of studies. Three important factors contributed to its development. In the first place, the reception of the entire corpus of Aristotelian writings took place during the twelfth century. Gerard of Cremona translated a great portion of the works of Artistotle as well as those of Galen and Hippocrates into Latin. Thus, the new universities had at hand a collection of works that offered a completely rational explanation of the universe in terms of natural causes. It must be recalled that Aristotle was a physician as well as a philosopher. Second, there occurred a gradual development of the idea of the official supervision and licensing of students. This was paralleled with a formalization of studies. And, finally, the involvement of the new mendicant orders, particularly Dominicans and Franciscans, in the faculties of the new universities. From among the friars came many of the great names in medieval medicine.

The first statute to establish that an exact curriculum had to be followed before degree was granted was issued in Paris in 1215. By the end of the fourteenth century, there were more than twenty-five institutions of higher learning granting the *jus docendi ubique*. In northern Europe, with the University of Paris as prototype, the faculty controlled the administration of the school. In the south, with the University of Bologna as the model, the school was controlled by the student body. While most of the newly founded universities had faculties of medicine as well as law and theology, the universities of Bologna and Montpelier were outstanding centers of medical studies.

Until the rise of the universities, the most renowned school of medicine in Europe was the famous school of Salerno. It was not organized along the same lines as the universities and seems to have had little influence upon them, but it was for several centuries considered the center of medical learning in the West. Before the nineteenth century, historians were wont to explain the presence of a medical school here to its proximity to the Arab world, but there were other reasons. Thanks to the salubrious climate and the presence of mineral springs, Salerno had enjoyed a reputation as a health resort during Roman times. There is no doubt that the tradition continued after the Germanic invasions. As early as the tenth century, chroniclers record this location as a home of physicians. Monks from the Benedictine monastery of Monte Cassino seem to have operated a hospital there as early as 820, but by the beginning of the eleventh century, the center was in lay hands. It was the Carthaginian-born Constantius Africanus (1020-1087) who first opened the center to the large body of Arabian literature that was to replace the neo-Latin sources used here. Constantius' most famous work was a translation of Arabian physician Ali ben El-Abbas, *Art of Medicine*, known in Latin Europe as the *Pantegni*. Under his influence, a number of works of anatomy were made available to the students, and efforts were made to introduce a regularized curriculum. During the twelfth century, the fame of Salerno had spread throughout all of Europe. It was known as the *Civitas Hippocratia*, or Hippocratic city. The first medical textbook on surgery, *Cyrurgia Rogerii*, the work of Roger of Polerno, who was an instructor there, appeared in 1170. Giles of Corbeil, whose work on uroscopy, *Carmina de Urinarum*, was used until the seventeenth century, was an alumnus of Salerno as was the English physician Gilbertus (1180-1250). The latter's *Compendium Medicinae*, containing one of the earliest descriptions of leprosy, was a standard work during the twelfth century. It was printed in Lyons as late as 1510.

It is significant in European history that the first official document to regulate the practice of medicine was issued in the environs of Salerno by Roger II of Sicily. This famous decree stipulates "that whoever from this time forth wishes to practice medicine (mederi voluerit) must present himself before our officials and judges and subject himself to their decisions. Whoever presumes to avoid this shall be constrained in prison and his goods confiscated. The purpose of this decree is to protect the subjects of our kingdom from being imperilled through the incompetence of physicians."

This legislation was again published in 1231 in the *Constitutiones Regni Sicili* of German Emperor Frederick I and expanded to include the establishment of medical fees. It stipulated free attendance to the indigent, the regulation of the purity and price of drugs, and the relations between physicians and pharmacists. No person was to be admitted to the study of medicine unless he had spent three years in the study of the trivium—logic, grammar, and rhetoric—and the study of the quadrivium—mathematics, geometry, astronomy, and music. Neither was he to teach in a school or exercise the curative craft until he had been examined by masters at Salerno or Naples, who were to make an inquiry into his knowledge of medicine and surgery.

Perhaps the most widely circulated medical tract of the medieval period was the *Regimen Sanitatis Salernitanum* of the School of Salerno. Probably written in Toledo, it is usually attributed to Arnold of Villanova, although its origins are obscure. More than three hundred editions of this medical poem have been printed, and it has been translated into all of the languages of modern Europe. Some sixteen English translations are recorded. The work, which is divided into ten sections, deals with hygiene, materia medica, anatomy, physiology, etiology, ectology, pathology, classification of diseases, and the practice of medicine. The following selection is based on a sixteenth-century English translation by Sir John Harington, inventor of the watercloset:

REGIMEN SANITATIS

White Muskadell, and *Candie* wine, and Greeke,
Do make men's wits and bodies grosse and fat;
Red wine doth make the voyce oft-time to seeke,
And hath a bidding qualitie to that;
Canarie, and *Madera,* both are like
To make one leane indeed: (but wot you what)
Who say they make one leane, would make one laffe
The meane, they make one leane upon a staffe.
Wine, women, Baths, by Art or Nature warme,
Us'd or abus'd do men much good or harme.

Sixe things, that here in order shall ensure,
Against all poysons have secret power,
Peare, Garlicke, Reddish-roots, Nuts, Rape, and Rue,
But *Garlicke* chiefe; for they that it devoure,
May drinke, & care not who their drinke do brew:
May walke in aires infected every houre.
Sith *Garlicke* then hath powers to save from death,
Beare with it though it make unsavory breath:
And scorne not *Garlicke,* like to some that thinke
It onley makes men winke, and drinke, and stinke.

Though ill favours do not breed infection,
Yet sure infection commeth most by smelling,
Who smelleth still perfumed, his complexion
Is not perfum'd by Poet *Martials* telling,

Yet for your lodging roomes give this direction,
In houses where you mind to make your dwelling,
That neere the same there be no evill sents
Of puddle-waters, or of excrements,
Let aire be cleere and light, and free from faults,
That come of secret passages and vaults.

If wine have over night a surfet brought,
A thing we wish to you should happen feel:
Then early in the morning drinke a draught,
And that a kind of remedie shall yeeld,
But gainst all surfets, vertues schoole hath taught
To make the gift of temperance a shield:
The better wines do breed the better humors,
The worse, are causes of unwholesome tumors.
In measure drinke, let wine be reipe, not thick.
But cleere and well alaid, and fresh and quicke.

The like advice we give you for your Beers,
We will it be not sowre, and yet be stale:
Well boild, of harty graine and old and cleare,
Nor drinke too much nor let it be too stale:
And as there be foure seasons in the yeere,
In each a severall order keepe you shall.
In *Spring* your dinner must not much exceed,
In *Summers* heate but little meate shall need:
In *Autumne* ware you eate not too much fruite:
With *Winters* cold full meates do fittest suite.

If in your drinke you mingle *Rew* with *Sage,*
All poyson is expeld by power of those,
And if you would withall Lusts heat asswage,
Adde to them two the gentle flowre of Rose:
Would not be sea-sicke when seas do rage,
Sage-water drinke with wine before he goes.
Salt, Garlicke, Parsly, Pepper, Sage, and Wine.
Make sawces for all meates both course and fine.
Of washing of your hands much good doth rise,
Tis wholesome, cleanely, and relieves your eyes.

Eate not your bread too stale, nor eate it hot,
A little Levened, hollow baked and light:
Not fresh of purest graine that can be got,
The crust breede choller bith of browne & white,

Yet let it be well bak't or eate it not,
How e're your taste therein may take delight.
Porke without wine is not so good to eate,
As Sheepe with wine, it medicine is and meate,
Tho Intrailes of a beast be not the best,
Yet some intrailes better than the rest.

Some love to drinke new wine not fully fin'd,
But for your health we wish that you drinke none,
For such to dangerous fluxes are inclin'd,
Besides, the Lees of wine doe breed the stone,
Some to drinke onely water are assign'd,
But such by our consent shall drinke alone.
For water and small beere we make no question,
Are enemies to health and good digestion:
And *Horace* in a verse of his rehearses,
That *Water-drinkers* never make good verses.

Salerno was later eclipsed by the new universities, especially Bologna and Montpelier. First mention of medical studies at Montpelier date from 1137, and by the second decade of the twelfth century, a degree-granting university had evolved.

A look at the books required for reading and lecture subjects decreed in 1340 shows a heavy predominance of Galen and Avicenna. The time required for a bachelor's degree in medicine was twenty-four months of attendance at lectures. Before obtaining a degree of bachelor of medicine, the candidate had to visit the sick with the instructor. The doctor's degree required five years if the candidate already possessed a master's; six years for other candidates. No person was allowed to practice until he had been examined and authorized by the bishop and his examiners. This was enforced under pain of excommunication.

Two of the most well known figures in the history of medieval medicine were associated with the University of Montpelier, Arnold of Villanova (1235–1311) and Guy de Chauliac (1300–68). Both were clerics and were educated by the Dominican friars. Arnold was the author of some sixty works dealing with philosophy, theology, and astrology as well as medicine. His reputed authorship of the *Regimen Sanitatis* attests to his fame. In addition to translating the works of Avicenna, on the heart, he composed a compendium dealing with surgery, gynecology, and toxicology. He is reputed to have introduced tinctures and brandy into *Pharmacopeia* and must be listed as a pioneer in the use of distilled spirits. Some historians consider that improved methods of distillation are the greatest single contribution of the Middle Ages to science. The earliest known account of the preparation of alcohol dates from the twelfth century.

Dominican friar Raymond Lull (1232–1315), who taught at Montpelier, advanced the process of distillation by introducing rectification by means of limestone and calix. Arnold used alcohol to extract medicine and recommended it as a drink. By the fifteenth century, the consumption of spirits, along with the traditional beer and wine, had advanced to the point where distillers had organized themselves into guilds. Improved methods of distillation also led to the preparation of nitric and sulphuric acids. Arnold was one of the first physicians in the West to recognize the importance of chemistry for medicine.

Guy de Chauliac, who was a student of Raymond Lull, is regarded by some as the father of surgery. After receiving a degree in medicine at the University of Montpelier, Chauliac attended the University of Bologna, which was particularly known for its excellence in surgical studies. It enjoyed a long tradition in dissection generated by the works of Taddeo Alderotte (1223–1303), William of Saliceto (1210–80), and Mondini de Luzzi (1270–1326). The latter, called the restorer of anatomy, wrote the first modern textbook, *Anathomia,* in 1316. This work, largely a compilation from Galen, was the standard text until the appearance of Vesalius' *Fabrica* in the sixteenth century. From Bologna, Chauliac transferred to the University of Paris, whose reputation rested to a great extent on the presence of Lanfranchi of Milan, author of a number of works on surgery. Lanfranchi is regarded as the inaugurator of a tradition of professionalism in surgery that distinguished French medicine until the nineteenth century. After completing his tour of the major centers of medical studies, Chauliac resided for a number of years in Lyon. From here, he was called to the residence of the popes in Avignon, where he acted as personal physician to Clement VI, Innocent VI, and Urban V. It was in his service of the popes that he composed his great work *Cyrgia Magna,* completed in 1363. This work was the authoritative text on surgery until the eighteenth century and was translated into French, Italian, Dutch, Spanish, German, and English. The excellence of the work lies in its treatment of surgery in the skull, thorax, and abdomen. In his treatment of hernia, he introduced the method of taxis, or manipulation to produce reduction, used until the nineteenth century. His treatment of cataracts by depression is a classic of medical literature.

This book also contains a firsthand account of the terrible plague, known as the Black Death, that ravaged Europe for several decades after 1347. It is estimated that one-third of Western Europe perished in what is now described as a combination of bubonic plague and pneumonia carried from India by the brown rat. As described by contemporaries, the disease was characterized by a swelling of lymphatic glands in the groin and armpit. Hence, the term bubonic. It is now known that the plague is caused by a bacillus, *Pasteurella pestis,* found in rats and other rodents and transmitted by the rat flea— *Xenopsylla Cheops.* Periodic epidemics of the plague affected Europe for the next three centuries.

The economic and social effects of the Black Death were catastrophic. The late Middle Ages witnessed a decline in population accompanied by gnawing tensions between the nobility, the peasants, and a growing urban population. Yet a number of benefits did result. In the first place, there was an increased concern over the nature of the transmission of disease. The ideas that specific diseases could be caught by contagion gradually developed. Leprosy had, of course, been recognized as contagious, and lepers had been segregated since the fifth century. Now it was often possible to diagnose this disease and isolate the patient in its early stages.

A realization that other diseases, smallpox, diphtheria, and typhoid, were transmitted also evolved, but it was not until the work of Fracastoro in the sixteenth century that any valid conclusions were reached.

The Black Death also made authorities aware of the need for preventative action. In northern Italy, where municipal governments first took root and where a larger urban population existed, cities began to enact legislation aimed at curtailing the movements of suspected carriers of contagion. Commissions of public health were established as early as 1343 in the Republic of San Marco and later in Lucca, Florence, and Perugia. Venetian-controlled Ragusa issued the first recorded law ordering a forty-day quarantine of all travelers arriving there from infected regions.

The period following the Black Death was also marked by a trend toward greater lay control of hospitals. The military hospital orders, founded during the first crusades, had of course done a great deal to promote hospital care. The Hospitalers, founded in the late eleventh century by merchants from Amelfi, had established a Christian hospital in Jerusalem dedicated to the Alexandrian saint, John the Almoner. Following the first crusade, the knights of the order operated excellently-managed hospitals in the port cities of Italy and France. The Teutonic Knights established hospitals for the indigent. The Order of Lazarus, founded in Jerusalem in 1220, maintained hospitals in France, Italy, England, Hungary, and Germany. It is estimated that by the thirteenth century there were more than nineteen thousand hospitals in western Europe, two thousand in France alone. Inmates included the poor, the sick, the old, the blind, lepers, and other unfortunates. As the urban middle class grew in the thirteenth century, and as the crusading fervor declined, hospitals came under the control and administration of municipalities. Like the medieval cathedral, the hospitals of this period were often astounding feats of architectural genius. Many of the late medieval hospitals were constructed, as were the cathedrals, in the form of a cross with the equal arms serving as long wards. The wards were lighted and ventilated by high windows in the vaulted roof. Recessed, partitioned cubicles provided privacy for patients. Ornamentation with richly carved woodwork was not uncommon. Although the patient's chances of recovering were remote, at least the atmosphere was more conducive to convalescence than in many of the modern hospitals.

It is generally agreed that medieval medicine remained static because it was overly speculative. Franciscan friar Roger Bacon (c. 1214–94) is one who advocated the investigative approach to learning. Stressing the important role of experimental science, Bacon taught at Oxford until 1257, when he was forced to give up public lectures because of his alleged defense of astrology. In his chief work, *Opus Majus,* he demonstrates an extraordinary knowledge of the science of optics, experimenting with plano-convex lenses. His description of the anatomy of the vertebrate eye and the optic nerve was far in advance of his age. Some of his recommendations have a timely ring. For example, he advocates a change of habitation for certain incorrigible malefactors, observing that a change of abode will bring about an amelioration of morals. His treatment of old age might be cited as an early approach to the science of geriatrics:

Another example can be given in the field of medicine regarding the lengthening of the life span, for which medicine has nothing to offer but a regimen of health. But a far longer life span is possible. In the beginning of the world, life was much longer, but by now this has been unduly shortened. Many men have thought that the answer to this problem lay in the heavens. They considered that the arrangement of the heavens was more exact in the earlier days, but as time passed things began to decline. They say that the stars were created in more perfect positions, that the stars have their dignities, and that therefore, with their many divers aspects, they should be more perfectly arranged. These men also say that the stars have gradually moved from their earlier, more perfect, positions, and in so doing, have imposed upon man a shortened life span, a boundary beyond which there is a state of rest. I will now address myself to the many contradictions and problems inherent in this idea.

Whether it can be proven or not, there is another reason which is simpler, more readily available and uncontradictable. We must strive for this reason, so that the splendor of experimental science might appear, and the way might be opened to the greatest of secrets, hidden in Aristotle's book on the regimen of life. Although the regimen of health should always be observed —in eating and drinking, asleep and awake, in motion or in rest, in loss or in retention, in the nature of the air and the passions of the mind—and although this should be done from the moment of birth, very few people follow them. In fact, only one physician in a thousand gives this matter the slightest attention. Very rarely does anyone pay sufficient heed to the rules of health. While almost no one follows them in his youth, many think of them when they are old and dying, for then they fear death and begin to think of their health. One cannot then apply a remedy because of weakened senses and powers, and lack of experience. Therefore, the fathers are weakened and sire weak sons with a tendency for an early death. By neglect of the rules of health, the sons are weakened, and therefore the next generation has a doubly weakened constitution. Then, in due time, the son, also, weakens himself by not following the rules of health. Thus, the weakness passes from father to son, growing greater, shortening the life span to that of the present day.

In addition to this accidental cause, there is another resulting from the disregard of morals. The powers of the soul are weakened by sins, making the normally competent control of the body impossible. Therefore, the powers of the body are lessened, and life is shortened. This decline is also passed from father to son, and so on through the generations. Because of these two natural causes, the longevity of man has, contrary to nature, been shortened from what it was in the beginning. It has been proven, moreover, that this excessive shortening of the life span has been retarded, and the span of life lengthened by many years by secret experiments. Since many authors have written about this, there must be a remedy for this apparently accidental shortening of life.

Since I have shown that the cause of a shortening of life is accidental, and therefore a remedy is possible, I will now return to the example that I have decided to give where the power of medicine fails. In this example, experiment supplies the defects in medicine which arise from the fact that medicine can give only the proper rules for health for those of all ages. Although eminent authors have not written adequately about the proper regimen for the aged, it has been possible for medicine to prescribe such a regimen. Such a regimen concerns the proper use of food and drink, of motion and rest, of sleep and wakefulness, of loss and retention, of the air and the control of the passions of the mind. If, in accordance with the feasibility of a proper regimen, a man were to follow, from birth, its precepts, he would reach the limits set by God and nature. However, since it is impossible for this regimen to be followed by anyone, and since almost none pays heed to it, particularly the young, and it is impossible for the aged to follow it, the accidents of old age come before the prime of life is reached, the age of beauty and strength. The prime of life is from forty-five to fifty years.

The accidents of old age and senility are: white hair, pallor, wrinkling of the skin, an excess of mucus, foul phlegm, inflammation of the eyes and a general injury to the sense organs, diminution of blood and the spirits, weakness of the body, both in motion and in breathing, the failure of both the animal and natural powers of the soul, sleeplessness, anger and disquietude of the mind, and finally, forgetfulness. The royal Hali says that old age is the home of forgetfulness, and Plato states that it is the mother of lethargy. Because of the lack of a proper health regimen, all of these accidents and many more come to men in the prime of life. That is, their life span is lengthened or shortened in accordance with the better or worse control they have exercised in the matter of their health, and in accordance with their constitution and their control of their morals. While the medical art does not furnish remedies for these corruptions that come from a lack of control and failures in regimen, medical authors confess that such remedies are possible, though not taught in the books. These remedies have always been hidden, not only from the physicians, but also from the scientists. They have only been known to the most noted, as described by Aristotle in the first book of the Topics, in the division of the probable. Not only are there possible remedies to prevent the conditions of old age from appearing during the prime of life and before their proper time, but these remedies can also retard the conditions of old age and senility so that they do not even appear at the ordinary time. If these conditions do come, they can be mitigated and moderated so that life may be prolonged beyond the limit set by a proper health regimen. However, while this first limit can be passed, the second, set by God and nature in accordance with the remedies retarding the accidents of old age and senility, cannot be passed.

Due to these two limits, the Scripture states, "Thou has set its bounds which cannot be passed." Therefore, while this first limit might rarely be passed, it is impossible to pass this ultimate limit. The proper health regimen, therefore, in so far as man possesses it, would only prolong life beyond the common, accidental limit. Man, because of his folly, does not protect for his own interest, and thus some have lived for many years beyond the common limit of life. A special regimen of remedies for retarding the common limit of life, not exceeded by the medical art, can prolong life much further. This is shown by Dioscorides, who states that there may be some medicine to protect man from the swiftness of old age, from colds and from the drying up of his members and with it, the life of man might be lengthened. In the Tengi, near the conclusion, Hali states that "those who have lived a long time have used medicines by which their life has been prolonged." In addition, in the second book of Canon, Avicenna states that "there is a medicine that settles and divides every constitution as it should be." However, medical authorities have not used those medicines, nor are they described in the medical texts. This is because, as has been previously stated, these writers pay attention only to the art of caring for the health, which, however, they do inefficiently. Learned men, devoted to experimental science, have studied these matters. They are influenced not only by their utility, but also by the action of animals, who avoid a premature death in many ways (i.e. the stag, the eagle, and the snake), and many other animals who prolong their life by natural action, as the authors state, and experience has shown. Guided by these examples, they believed that God himself had granted this power to the beasts for the instruction of mortal man. Therefore, they watched the animals so that they might learn the power of the herbs, stones, metals and other things by which they improve their bodies in apparently miraculous ways. They do this in the same manner as we gather information, with the utmost certainty, from the books of Pliny, Solinus, Avicenna on Animals, Tullius on the Divine Nature, from the philosophy of Artephius and from other books and various authors and from people who have experience in this matter. Recently in Paris, there was a scientist who took a snake and cut it into small portions, except for the skin of the belly, which he left intact. The snake crept to a certain herb and by its touch was cured. Encouraged by the examples of animals, and since human reason is superior to the wisdom of animals, scientists have discovered better and greater means.

This wisdom was granted to the world through the first men, Adam and his sons, who received from God special knowledge so that they might prolong their lives. We learn from Aristotle in the book of Secrets that God most high and glorious has prepared a means and a remedy for tempering the humors, preserving the health, for acquiring things which will combat the ills of old age and to retard and mitigate such evils. These remedies God revealed to his saints and prophets, and to certain others, such as the patriarch, whom He chose and enlightened with the spirit of divine wisdom. (*Opus Majus, Scientia Experimentalis,* Cap. XII, Ex. II)

The medieval world, while it struggled to reclaim what had been lost with the collapse of Hellenistic culture, did contribute at least in a general way to medical science. By organizing and certifying medical studies, it made possible a cooperative effort in medical research. It fostered the idea that the aim of science was to harness the forces of nature and use them for the benefit of mankind. Finally, the medieval mind realized that no particular scientific theory was irreplaceable. The dialectics of the schoolmen were based on the premise that by doubting we come to questioning and with frequent questioning we arrive at the truth.

As in every age, the medieval period produced its share of literary criticism of the medical profession. Petrarch, the father of Renaissance letters, constantly chides the medical profession for its servile adherence to Arabian textbooks, mendacity, and pomposity. In a series of letters to a well-known physician of Sienna, Franciscus di Sieno, he expresses his disdain for doctors of medicine, citing among other instances the inscription on a tombstone: "the multitude of a physician killed me." In a letter to Boccacio, he describes the splendid attire worn by physicians in public, royal scarlet embellished with priceless gems, and gilded spurs. There is, he remarks, a certain similarity between the guild of physicians on parade and the triumphal victory march of a returning army because both can be credited with the slaughter of five thousand men. The only difference is that the medical murders were perpetrated on fellow citizens by unarmed persons dressed in togas and huddled behind monumental piles of drugs. A more congenial description of a medieval doctor can be found in Geoffrey Chaucer's *Canterbury Tales:*

> *With us ther was a Doctour of Phisik;*
> *In al this world ne was ther noon hym lik,*
> *To speke of phisik and of surgerye,*
> *For he was grounded in astronomye.*
> *He kepte his pacient a ful greet deel*
> *In houres by his magyk natureel.*
> *Wel koude he fortunen the ascendent*

Of his ymages for his pacient.
He knew the cause of everich maladye,
Were it of hoot, or coold, or moyste, or drye,
And where they engendred, and of what humour.
He was a verray, parfit praktisour:
The cause yknowe, and of his harm the roote,
Anon he yaf the sike man his boote.
Ful redy hadde he his apothecaries
To sende hym drogges and his letuaries.
For ech of hem made oother for to wynne—
Hir frendshipe nas nat newe to bigynne.
Wel knew he the olde Esculapius,
And Deyscorides, and eek Rufus,
Olde Ypocras, Haly, and Galyen,
Serapion, Razis, and Avycen,
Averrois, Damascien, and Constantyn,
Bernard, and Gatesden, and Gilbertyn.
Of his diete mesurable was he,
For it was of no superfluitee,
But of greet norissyng and digestible.
His studie was but litel on the Bible.
In sangwyn and in pers he clad was al,
Lyned with taffata and with sendal;
And yet he was but esy of dispence;
He kepte that he wan in pestilence.
For gold in phisik is a cordial,
Therefore he lovede gold in special.

5

The Renaissance

"AT THE SOUND of the word 'Renaissance' the dreamer of past beauty sees purple and gold. A festive world is bathed in mild clarity, rustling with sonorous tones. People move with grace and solemnity, untroubled by the distress of time and the beckonings of eternity. Everything is one ripe, full exuberance." With these words, Dutch historian Johan Huizinga introduced a famous lecture entitled "The Problem of the Renaissance," which has during the past half-century engendered a plethora of studies and monographs on the nature of the Renaissance. Some historians now deny its very existence; others question its impact on Western culture. Yet, for many, the problem of the Renaissance is a simple one. The Renaissance was the emergence of individualism, the awakening of the urge to beauty, the triumph of secularism and *joie de vivre,* and the conquest of mundane reality by the mind.

Influenced by Swiss historian Jakob Burckhardt's *Kunst und Kultur der Renaissance in Italien* (1860), there is a general belief that this period witnessed the birth of the modern world and the self-discovery of man, who had long been imprisoned by the religious asceticism and intolerant authority of the Middle Ages. It was the rediscovery of the cosmos and the individual. The notion of individualism as the key mark of the Renaissance was especially popular during the late nineteenth century, and finds its present support in the egalitarian philosophies of our own time.

Yet as is the case with practically all other historical periods, the interpretation of the Renaissance underwent notable changes in the past fifty years. Historians now question not only the traditional ear-

84

marks of the age but also its overall effects on European culture. Much of this questioning results from continuing attacks on the Burckhardtian thesis, with its strong classical-rational and Hegelian overtones. As usually understood, the thesis maintained that the basic elements of modern civilization first appeared in a rudimentary form in fifteenth and sixteenth-century Italy and spread to the northern countries.

The assault on this thesis was based on nationalism, religious romanticism, and the new social and economic sciences. Carl Neumann, one of Burckhardt's students and his biographer, rejecting his master's claim to the classical element in the fourteenth-century revival, stressed that the culture of antiquity had perdured in the Byzantine world with no similar results, no *vita nuova*. The three basic elements of Western culture as seen by Neumann, antiquity, Christianity, and *"Germanentum,"* did not amalgamate in the Greek world. It was this latter element—Germanism—that provided Western culture with its specific coloring. The mixing of these three elements gave Western man a new soul *(eine neue Seele)*. Subsequent German writers traced a direct Lombardic or Gothic descent for all the illuminati of the Italian Renaissance from Dante to Michaelangelo. Not to be outdone in chauvinism, French and Belgian historians assembled proof for the French and Burgundian origins of the movement. Seeing "realism" rather than individualism as a term best summarizing the Renaissance, art historian Louis Courajod offered the thesis that Gothic architecture regenerated independent of Italian influence by turning to absolute naturalism. It was from this regeneration that the Renaissance sprang. Instead of flowering northward, the Renaissance now appeared to have been a southward influx of Nordic and Gallic achievements into "barbarian" Italy.

The medievalist added a new dimension to the ever-changing concept of the Renaissance when Charles Homer Haskins in the United States and Franz von Bezhold in Germany discovered a Renaissance in the twelfth century.

Economists and sociologists have found that capitalism and civic spirit were the elements that differentiated the "Renaissance man" from his medieval antecedents. For sociologist Alfred von Martin, for example, who combines Marx with Burckhardt, the humanist movement of the Renaissance was a weapon of the bourgeosie against the old aristocratic-ecclesiastic social order of the Middle Ages.

Out of this ever-growing mass of interpretation there has gradually emerged a view of the Renaissance that has stripped it of the uniqueness and status ascribed to it by Burckhardt. In the words of Wallace K. Fergeson: "The Renaissance was essentially an age of transition containing much that was still medieval, much that was recognizably modern, also, much that, because of the mixture of medieval and modern elements was peculiar to itself and was responsible for its contradictions and contrasts and its amazing vitality."

Hence, the Renaissance was not merely the revival of classicism; it was the advent of an entirely new culture, a new way of life that found its roots centuries in the past and that had been long developing in the Mediterranean world before its fullest expression in fifteenth-century Italy. As a new culture, it was characterized by civic responsibility, individualism, a strict observation of nature, and a critical mentality. It was a shift from a logical to a more psychological outlook that was aesthetically oriented. Like the Hellenistic world, which it so slavishly imitated, it possessed an urban culture. Only in Italy, where the ancient cities had never disappeared, could a civilization characterized by a vigorous civic life and intense political and economic rivalry revive. Florence, especially, became the birthplace of this Western culture in the three centuries from Petrarch to Galileo. It was rich in movement, rivalry, and creative power as no other city in western Europe. Here business acumen and mechanical science combined to create techniques based on a knowledge of natural laws.

Like politics and culture, medicine in the Renaissance also was in a period of transition. There was much that was medieval and a great deal that was novel, but for the most part a combination of the two predominated.

The rediscovery of the classical world gave a new dimension to the medical literature of the period, and the newly invented art of printing helped to disseminate a body of medical writings in the original Greek and Latin. By the middle of the sixteenth century, most of the classical medical writings that we now possess had appeared in print. The *De Medicina* of Celsus, discovered in 1443, was published at Florence in 1478 and was widely acclaimed because of the purity of its style and its historical content. Celsus' work was of particular importance because it provided the medical world with a new Latin nomenclature, thus replacing the Latinized Arabic words so much a part of medieval medical literature. Many commonplace terms, such as abdomen, anus, cartilage, radius, scrotum, tibia, tonsil, uterus, and vertebra, were introduced.

The replacement of Arabic terms, however, was a long and drawn-out process. Conservatives retained the older vocabulary well into the seventeenth century. The aphorisms of Hippocrates were translated by Niccolo Leonceno in Italy and François Rabelais (1494?–1553) in France. A critical edition of the Greek text of Hippocrates was completed in 1595 by Antonius Foes of Metz. In England, Thomas Linacre (1460?–1524) translated important works of Galen. It was not until the twentieth century, with the creation in Germany of commissions to publish critical editions of the ancient Greek and Latin authors (Corpus Medicorum Graecorum in Berlin and the Corpus Medicorum Latinorum in Leipzig), that the work begun by the Renaissance humanists was renewed on a large scale.

The printing of more reliable medical works in Venice, Basel, Lyons, and Paris now provided students with cheap and reliable texts and eventually weakened the hold of the Arabian medieval authorities. At the same time, the universities began to adapt the curriculum to the new sources by eliminating many of the traditional medical studies, especially those of Avicenna, and by introducing clinical and bedside teaching. Another result of the new learning was the development of medical botany. Following the example of Padua, which in 1553 established a chair of botany, special botanical gardens were established at the universities of Leiden, Leipzig, Paris, and Heidelberg before the end of the century. Interest in botany was to climax in the eighteenth century in the work of the Swedish physician Carl von Linnaeus (1707–78), whose Septima Naturae, published in 1735, still forms the basis for plant classification.

A new direction in anatomical studies was taken when professors actually carried out the dissections themselves. Students were given the opportunity for closer observation with the introduction of anatomical theaters, or amphitheaters, wherein the instructor would demonstrate on an elevated stage. In some cases, the theaters would accommodate as many as five hundred spectators.

Although the "new learning" in medicine was hailed as a rebirth, it had the fatal flaw of perpetuating the errors of Greek medicine. The establishment of new "Hippocratic" and "Galenic" schools was in a certain sense a disservice to the new discoveries that occurred during the period.

Among those who shared in the enthusiasm for the new Greek medicine and contributed to its implementation was English priest and physician Thomas Linacre. Born at Canterbury in about 1460, he entered Oxford in 1480 and four years later was elected a Fellow of All Souls College, where he devoted himself to the study of Greek. During the late 1480s, he traveled to Italy, where he studied under the leading humanists in Florence and Rome. At the urging of Hermolaus Barbarous, Linacre enrolled at the medical school of Padua and received a medical degree in 1496. Returning to England, he was entrusted by Henry VII with the care of his ailing son Arthur. Upon the accession of Henry VIII in 1509, Linacre was appointed personal physician to the king. Among his other prominent patients were Sir Reynold Broy, royal treasurer; Cardinal Wolsey; and the Archbishop of Canterbury, William Warham. Linacre's position of influence at court and Henry's personal interest in medicine led, in 1513, to the adoption of the Medical Act. The two sponsors of this bill, "the first attempt to regulate medicine in England," were the bishop of London and the dean of St. Paul's, the educator John Colet. At Linacre's urging these two men sponsored the bill and guided it to enactment. The act provided that no one who had not attended Oxford or Cambridge could practice medicine within seven miles of London without being examined, approved, and admitted by the bishop of London, assisted by four qualified physicians. Outside the city, the bishop of each diocese was in charge of examining and approving doctors.

Later, in 1518, this act was supplemented by the establishment of the College of Physicians, later called the Royal College of Physicians. The college was neither a medical school nor an institution for learning in the modern sense; essentially a governing body, it was composed of six Elects, or Directors, who chose Linacre as their first president. Once again, the college decreed that only graduates of Oxford or Cambridge would be allowed to practice medicine until examined and approved, now by the president of the college and the Elects. In this way, it was made certain that future physicians would be educated at the universities and also that they would be examined by the highest ranking doctors of the kingdom. In addition, it required that apothecaries have their medicines examined and approved by the Elects of the College. In 1522, the jurisdiction of the college was extended to include the entire realm.

One of Linacre's patients and close associates in the editing of the texts was the most famous scholar of the period, Erasmus of Rotterdam (c. 1466–1536). Known to this day for his famous *Praise of Folly,* Erasmus published a lesser known work, *The Praise of Medicine,* in which he demonstrates his interest in, and wide knowledge of, the history of medicine. Although the main target of his criticism was the medieval church, he did not spare the medical profession, as the following excerpt from his colloquy, *The Funeral,* indicates:

PHAEDUS: First hear about George, then. The moment unmistakable signs of death appeared, the company of physicians who had long attended the patient began to demand their fees, hiding their feeling of hopelessness about his life.

MARCUS: How many doctors were there?

PHAEDUS: Sometimes ten, sometimes twelve; never fewer than six.

MARCUS: Enough to kill even a healthy man!

PHAEDUS: When they had their money, they warned the relatives confidentially that death was not far off; that they should look to his spiritual welfare, for there was no hope of his physical safety. And the patient was warned courteously by his close friends to entrust his body to God's care, concerning himself only with that which belonged to making a good end. When he heard this, George stared at the physicians in wild surmise, as though indignant at being deserted by them. They retorted that they were physicians, not gods; that what their skill could do had been performed; but that no medicine could prevail against destiny. After this, they went into the next bedroom.

MARCUS: What? They lingered even after they were paid?

PHAEDUS: They had disagreed completely over what sort of disease it was. One said dropsy; another, tympanites; another, an intestinal abscess—each one named a different ailment. And during the whole time they were treating the patient they quarrelled violently about the nature of his malady.

MARCUS: Lucky patient meanwhile!

PHAEDUS: To settle their dispute once for all, they requested through his wife that they be permitted later to perform an autopsy on the body—quite a compliment, that, and done customarily as a mark of respect in the case of eminent persons. Furthermore, it would help save many lives and would increase George's accumulation of merits. Last of all, they promised to buy a trental of Masses at their own expense for the repose of his soul. This request met with opposition, to be sure, but was finally granted, thanks to their flattery of his wife and relations. Business disposed of, the medical congress adjourned, because it's not right, they say, for those whose job it is to save life to look on at death or to attend funerals.

Two important facets of the Renaissance world, the development of new techniques and weaponry in warfare, especially the use of gunpowder, and the discovery of new lands had a definite effect on the course of medical history. The invention of gunpowder was of Chinese origin and dates to the first century B.C. It was known in the West by the thirteenth century. The first firearms appeared a century later, and by the Hundred Years' War, cannon were being used by both the French and the English. With new methods of boring cast iron or bronze guns, the sixteenth century witnessed a great advance in the use of artillery, the large-scale use of which was introduced with the massive French invasion of Italy in 1494. A force of more than thirty thousand represented the largest army to invade the peninsula since the time of Hannibal. During the first half of the sixteenth century, the Imperial and Spanish armies of Charles V were engaged in five wars against France with peripheral engagements against the Turks and German Protestants. The size of land armies was paralleled in naval operation. Charles V landed a force of thirty-five thousand men against Tunis in 1535. The battles of Lepanto and the Armada involved unprecedented numbers of military personnel at sea.

It was against this background of increased warfare that the father of modern surgery, Ambroise Paré (1510–90), made his mark in medical history. Arriving in Paris in 1532 from provincial Brittany, he worked for a number of years as a dresser at the Hôtel Dieu. With the renewal of the war with the German Empire, he joined the troops of Francis I and saw at firsthand the dreadful effects of gunshot wounds. The usual treatment for such wounds was cauterization with burning oil. Running out of oil, Paré was forced to treat them with a mixture of egg yolks, oil of roses, and turpentine. He discovered that the wounds so treated were much better than those that had been burned and resolved never again to burn men wounded with gunshot. Returning to Paris in 1541, he was urged by the anatomist Jacques Dubois to write a book on the treatment of battlefield wounds. In 1545, there appeared the first of some twenty books he was to publish. Because Paré was not schooled in Latin, the work was written in the vernacular and entitled *La Méthode de Traicter les playes faictés par hacquebutes (The Method of Treating Wounds Made by Arquebuses)*. Before the end of the century, the book was translated into other languages and used by surgeons of most European armies.

In 1552, Paré was appointed to the court of Henry II and two years later given recognition by the Surgeon Confraternity and made a Master of Surgery. His most famous work, *A General History of Surgery*, appeared in 1563. The successors of Henry II, whom he attended on his deathbed, Francis II and Charles IX, retained him as court surgeon. It was this royal patronage that saved Paré from assassination during the notorious Massacre of St. Bartholomew's Night. He was suspected of harboring Huguenot sympathizers.

In addition to his success in abolishing cautery, Paré also reintroduced the practice of ligature, which had been lost since the Roman era. His works contain instructions on the use of artificial limbs and eyes. He strongly advocated the use of the truss for hernia and was the first to suggest that syphilis caused aneurysm. There is a great deal of truth in the observation that Paré, the self-educated doctor, is the father of modern surgery.

As with surgery, the wars of the sixteenth century provided pathology with a fertile field for widening knowledge. The mass movement of troops, the cramped and unhygienic conditions of the camps, and the breeding grounds provided by the stabling of horses made the plague the scourge of sixteenth-century Europe. Epidemics of the bubonic plague are recorded in 1509, 1514, 1526, 1560, and 1576. Typhus reached epidemic proportions in Italy in 1505 and again in 1528. In Spain, the diseases wiped out thousands in 1539 and 1572. Germany and Hungary both show records of typhus, which the Imperial troops called *"morbus hungaricus."* Venereal diseases, especially syphilis, increased throughout most of western Europe.

Italian-born physician Jerome Fracastoro (1478–1553), whose poem *Syphylidus* provided the nomenclature for syphilis, was descended from a well-established family of Veronese patricians and educated at the University of Padua. His rise in the academic world was meteoric. In 1501, he was appointed lecturer in logic at the University of Padua. His early interest in philosophy was to bear fruit later in a number of metaphysical tracts, *De Intellectione (On the Intellect), De Anima (On the Soul),* and *De Poetica (A Commentary on Aristotle's Poetics).* There is reason to believe that during this period Fracastoro came under the influence of his fellow-student Nicholas Copernicus (1473–1543). The Polish cleric studied at Padua from 1501 to 1506 and had already begun his lifelong preoccupation that was to culminate in his epoch-making work, *De Revolutionibus Caelistium Orbium (Concerning the Revolutions of the Celestial Bodies).* He later practiced medicine in his native Poland and wrote a number of works on the subject.

Like Copernicus, Fracastoro showed an interest in astronomy and cosmology. In 1538, he published a work entitled *Homocentrica sine de Stellis,* in which he sought, like Copernicus, to improve Aristotle's and Ptolemy's system of astronomy. The work attempted to conceive of the universe as a system of concentric spheres representing planetary motions in numerical detail by means of geometrical devices. His interests also included geography and geology.

Fracastoro's career as a lecturer at Padua was short lived. The League of Cambrai, formed in 1508 by Pope Julius II, united the German Emperor Maximillian and the kings of Spain, France, and Hungary against the Republic of Venice. Situated in Venetian territory, the University of Padua was forced to close its doors. The city of Verona was occupied by German troops, and Fracastoro was forced to flee. He spent most of his later career at his estate on the shores of Lake Garda. Although he practiced medicine, he turned more and more to the patronage of such high-ranking ecclesiastics as Pietro Bembo, secretary to Pope Leo X; Gian Matteo Giberti, bishop of Verona and secretary to Giulio de Medici; and Allesandro Farnese, secretary of state for Paul III. This clerical patronage culminated in Fracastoro's appointment as official physician to the Council of Trent, in 1546.

Fracastoro first achieved international fame in 1530 with the publication of his poem entitled *Syphilidus sive de Morbo Gallico (Syphilis or the French Disease).* The work consists of three books of thirteen hundred Latin Vergilian hexameters and is a potpourri of classical mythology, Renaissance cosmology, and contemporary history set partially in the New World. Syphilis, who does not appear until the third book, is a creation of Fracastoro's imagination. He appears as a shepherd to King Alcithous of Haiti. The former is afflicted with a terrible disease sent by the god Apollo. The natives of the island call the affliction syphilis.

Curiously, Fracastoro does not identify the disease with sexual morality but sees it as a result of widespread blasphemy. Nor does he subscribe to the popular belief that the disease originated in the New World. There is, as he sees it, nothing new about the malady. He attributes its current epidemic nature to the French invasion of Italy, hence the name, French Disease. The disease is found all over Europe and parts of Asia and Africa. Among the cures that he recommends are dictamon, or decoctions of cedar as a purgative, mercury, and above all the use of guaiac, derived from the huyacus tree, which grows in the Lesser Antilles.

Although Fracastoro achieved immediate fame as a poet with the publication of *Syphilidus,* his most important work, *De Contagiosis Moribus (On Contagious Diseases),* appeared sixteen years later. In his treatment of contagion, he described what many students of medical history consider to be a major breakthrough in the history of medicine. The work contains the first scientific statement of the true nature of contagion, of infection, of disease germs, and of the modes of transmission of infectious disease. He describes contagion as a corruption that develops in the substance of a combination, passes from one thing to another, and is originally caused by infection of the imperceptible particles. These germs are described as particles too small to be perceived by the senses but that, given the appropriate "media," are capable of reproduction and thus of infecting the surrounding tissue. Here, according to a number of authorities, is an account of the nature of disease germs that anticipates the later discoveries of Kircher, Leeuwenhoek, Koch, and Pasteur. Fracastoro believed that the pathogenic units were colloidal in nature; for if they were not viscous or glutinous by nature, they could not be transmitted through the atmosphere.

Fracastoro also observed that germs become pathogenic through the action of heat and that in order to produce disease they undergo only metabolic change. In addition to a general description of contagion, the book also treats poxes, pestilent fevers, typhus, rabies, elephantiasis, various cutaneous infections, and syphilis. Here is how he defines pestilent fever:

If, then, we permit ourselves to define pestilent fever, we shall say: *It is a fever of foul and deep-seated putrefaction; it contains germs of the most acute contagion per se; hence it is a deadly disease, and is contagious for another person.* This, then, and not putrefaction of the heart or its contents, is the essential characteristic of a pestilent fever. Not that there is any reason why the putrefaction should not be carried to them, also, especially if there exists an analogy between them and the putrefaction. But whether this be the case or not, it is not the essential characteristic of the plague, though perhaps it is characteristic of a more violent form of plague which is more quickly fatal.

But the thing that is essential and as they say formal, is that it is a fever which contains in itself the germs of death-dealing contagion. For these reasons, fevers that are caused by poisons, though deadly, are not pestilent, since they are not contagious. For they lack that formal and essential characteristic of the plague.

There is a prophetic and timely note in his observation that syphilis will pass away and be extinguished, to be born again and seen by our descendants.

Fracastoro was neither the first nor the last Renaissance physician to write on syphilis. Antonio Benivieni, a Florentine physician, described the disease in 1496, and a year later, Niccolo Leonecino published a work on the Gallican Disease in which he claimed that syphilis had been known in antiquity.

One of the most controversial figures of Renaissance medicine is the eccentric Theophrastus Bombastus von Hohenheim (1493–1541), or, as he is more commonly known, Paracelsus. The son of a German physician, he spent most of his youth in Villach, Switzerland. After attending a number of medical schools and studying with the controversial Benedictine abbot, Basil Valentine, the "father of antimony," he finally received a medical degree at the University of Ferrara. Paracelsus spent the next several years as a surgeon in a variety of armies in the Low Country, Scandinavia, and Italy. His experiences there bore fruit in his instructions for the treatment of bullet and arrow wounds in his *Grosse Wundartzney,* published in 1536. He also wrote books on syphilis, astrology, and philosophy, most of which were not published until long after his death. He was eventually given a chair of medicine at Basel.

In 1527, Paracelsus publicly burned the revered *Canon of Medicine* of Avicenna, thus launching an attack on the traditional medieval medical authorities. (Public book burning, inspired by Luther's celebrated incineration of the books of canon law, had become a fine art by the middle of the sixteenth century.) Moreover, Paracelsus' teaching methods did not endear him to the faculty, and he left Basel after a year and continued wandering. There is evidence that he suffered from an endocrine disorder, probably goiter, which was so common among the inhabitants of the Alpine region. Both in his lectures and in his writing, he exhibited a pomposity that was to make his middle name, Bombast, synonymous with ostentation.

Like other mavericks in the history of medicine, Paracelsus' contribution to science remains controversial. Although he was considered a quack by his contemporaries, modern interest has resulted in a cult-like revival of his achievements. The Paracelsus Society, founded in 1942, views him as the discoverer of vitamins, the forerunner of the Swiss Red Cross, and the father of iatrochemistry. In his works on mining diseases, he focused attention on the ill effects of fumes produced from smelters and describes mercury and arsenic poisoning. Because he experimented with sulphuric ether, some claim that he is the father of anesthesia. There is little doubt that his observations in work-related illnesses, especially in mines, have a timely ring, and he can be regarded as a pioneer in the area of environmental medicine. With the introduction of such chemicals as copper sulfate and potassium sulfate, Paracelsus marked a trend away from the Galenic world of herbal medicaments to modern chemical pharmacology. Yet his preoccupation with the occult and esoterica have shadowed whatever his real achievements may have been.

Most historians agree that the real advances made in medicine during the Renaissance were in the area of anatomy, a step that marked the superiority of Western medicine in the following centuries. Two figures dominate the progress made in this area, both northern Europeans and both associated with the school of Padua, the Belgian-born Andreas Vesalius (1514–64) and the Englishman William Harvey (1578–1657).

Vesalius can be regarded as the *Wunderkind* of his age, as his celebrated work *De Humanis Corporis Fabrica (On the Makeup of the Human Body)* was published in 1543, when he was only twenty-eight years of age. Its appearance coincided with the publication of Copernicus' *De Revolutionibus Caelestium Orbium,* and both were to mark a new era in the history of Western civilization. The family of Vesalius had for several generations been associated medically with the imperial Hapsburgs. Andreas' great-grandfather was physician to the wife of the Emperor Maximilian, his father was apothecary to the Belgian-born Emperor Charles V, and he himself became personal physician to the same emperor in 1544.

In many ways, Vesalius was the product of the classical learning of Renaissance humanism. The flawless Latin of his major work ranks him with the great authors of antiquity. His command of Greek showed that he was one of the most accomplished scholars of his day.

Some credit for this must be given to his teacher at the University of Paris, the humanist Jacobus Sylvius, who was later to achieve fame as a neo-Galenist. Vesalius matriculated at the University of Paris medical school at the age of seventeen. After several years in Paris, he returned to the Low Country and attended the University of Louvain, where he published his first work, *Paraphrases,* a paraphrase of the ninth book of Rhazes, probably as a thesis for his bachelor's degree at Paris.

In 1537, Vesalius was appointed to the chair of surgery and anatomy at the University of Padua, where he was to remain until 1542. Here he prepared and published his two most important medical works, the *Tabulae Anatomicae De Humanis Corporis Fabrica* and the *Epitome.* The *Fabrica* is extremely important in the history of anatomy; it proved that much of the time-honored anatomy of Galen was false because it was based on nonhuman parts. Unlike previous works on the subject, the *Fabrica* was based on dissections of human bodies from the years 1539 to 1543, often with the connivance of the local judge of the criminal court who delayed executions to accommodate Vesalius' investigations. The cry of the Renaissance humanist, *ad fontes,* was carried out literally by the anatomist Vesalius—to human bodies.

The *Fabrica* consists of seven books: the first dealing with the bones; the second, the muscles; the third, the vascular system; the fourth, the nervous system; the fifth, the abdominal viscera; the sixth, the heart and lungs; and the seventh, the brain. The work is profusely illustrated with anatomical figures attributed to Calcar (Joannes Stephanus), a student of Titian.

In the following passage, Vesalius explains to his patron, Charles V, why he wrote his famous work:

A number of obstacles, most gracious Emperor Charles, stand in the way of those investigating the scientific arts so that they are not accurately or fully learned, and I believe furthermore that no little loss occurs through the very great separation that has taken place between those disciplines that complement one another for the fullest comprehension of a single art; even much more the very capricious division by practitioners of an art into separate specialties so that those who set the limits of the art for themselves tenaciously grasp one part of it while other things which are in fact very closely related are cast aside. Consequently, they never demonstrate excellence and never attain their proposed end but constantly fall away from the true foundation of that art.

I will say nothing of the arts but I shall speak briefly of that which concerns the health of mankind; indeed, of all the arts the genius of man has discovered it is by far the most beneficial and of prime necessity, although difficult and laborious. Nothing was able to plague it more than when at one time, and especially after the Gothic invasions and the reign of Mansor, King of Persia —under whom the Arabs lived, as was proper, on terms of familiarity with the Greeks—medicine began to be maimed by the neglect of that primary instrument, the hand, so that [its uses] were relegated to ordinary persons wholly untrained in the disciplines subserving the art of medicine. Once there were three medical sects, that is, Dogmatic, Empirical, and Methodical, but their members consulted the whole art as the means of preserving health and driving away sicknesses. All the thoughts of each sect were directed toward this goal and three methods were employed: The first was a regimen of diet, the second the use of drugs, and the third the use of the hands. Except for this last, the other methods clearly indicate that medicine is the addition of things lacking and the withdrawal of superfluities; as often as we resort to medicine it displays its usefulness in the treatment of sickness, as time and experience teach, and its great benefit to mankind. This triple method of treatment was equally familiar to the physicians of each sect, and those using their own hands according to the nature of the sickness used no less effort in training them than in establishing a theory of diet or in understanding and compounding drugs.

In addition to the other books so perfectly composed by the divine Hippocrates, this is very clearly demonstrated in those *On the function of the physician, On fractures of bones,* and *On dislocations of joints and similar ailments.* Furthermore, Galen, after Hippocrates the prince of medicine, in addition to his occasional boast that the care of the gladiators of Pergamum was entrusted solely to him, and that although age was already weighing him down it did not please him that the monkeys he was to dissect should be skinned by slaves, frequently assures us of his pleasure in the employment of his hands and how zealously, like other Asiatic physicians, he used them. Indeed, none of the other ancients was so concerned that the treatment made with the hands, as well as that performed by diet and drugs, be handed down to posterity.

Especially after the devastation of the Goths when all the sciences, formerly so flourishing and fittingly practiced, had decayed, the more fashionable physicians, first in Italy in imitation of the old Romans, despising the use of the hands, began to relegate to their slaves those things which had to be done manually for their patients and to stand over them like architects. Then when, by degrees, others who practiced true medicine also declined those unpleasant duties—not, however, reducing their fees or dignity—they promptly degenerated from the earlier physicians, leaving the method of cooking and all the preparation of the patients' diet to nurses, the composition of drugs to apothecaries, and the use of the hands to barbers. And so in the course of time the art of treatment had been so miserably distorted that certain doctors assuming the name of physicians have arrogated to themselves the prescription of drugs and diet for obscure diseases, and have relegated the rest of medicine to those whom they call surgeons but consider scarcely as slaves. They have shamefully rid themselves of what is the chief and most venerable branch of medicine, that which based itself principally upon the investigation of nature—as if there were any other; even today (this part of the art) is exercised among the Indians, especially by the kings, and in Persia by law of inheritance it is handed down to the children as once the whole art was by the Asclepiads. The Thracians, with many other nations, cultivate and honor it very highly almost to the neglect of that other part of the art, the prescription of drugs. This the Romans once proscribed from the state considering it delusive and destructive of mankind, and of no benefit to nature since, although seeking to aid nature while it is wholly concerned in an attempt to throw off the sickness, drugs frequently make matters worse and distract nature from its proper function.

It is because of this that so many jibes are frequently cast at physicians and this very holy art is mocked, although part of it, which those trained in the liberal arts shamefully permit to be torn away from them, could readily adorn it forever with special lustre. When Homer, that source of genius, declared that a physician is more distinguished than a host of other men, and, with all the poets of Greece, celebrated Podalirius and Machaon, those divine sons of Aesculapius were praised not so much because they dispelled a little fever or something else of slight consequences, which nature alone could cure more readily without the aid of a physician than with it, nor because they yielded to the summons of men in obscure and desperate affections, but because they devoted themselves especially to the treatment of luxations, fractures, wounds, and other solutions of continuity and fluxions of blood, and because they freed Agamemnon's noble warriors of javelins, darts, and other evils of that sort which are the peculiar accompaniment of wars, and which always require the careful attention of the physician. *(Fabrica, Praefatio)*

In 1564, Vesalius traveled to the Holy Land on a pilgrimage from which he never returned. Having visited the holy places in Palestine, he died suddenly on the island of Zante during the return trip.

If Vesalius laid the foundations for modern scientific anatomical investigation, it can be said that William Harvey placed the keystone in position. Harvey was born in Folkestone, England, in 1578. Following six years of study at the University of Cambridge, he entered the University of Padua in 1599 to study under Fabricius of Aquapendente, who was well-grounded in Latin and Greek, especially the works of Aristotle. The excellent quality of anatomical studies inaugurated at Padua earlier in the century by Vesalius had been maintained by his succcessors Realdus Columba, Gabriel Fallopia, Hieronymus Fabricius, and Giulio Casserio.

Columba (1516–59) is of special interest as a precursor of Harvey because he wrestled with the problem left unsolved by Vesalius: how the blood got from the right ventricle of the heart to the left. As we have seen, Galen postulated that blood was formed in the liver, where it was imbued with the "natural spirits" of the source of life and nourishment. From the liver, this venous blood, as it was called, was carried to all parts of the body, where each part retained whatever amount was required, with fresh supplies available from the liver. Most of the blood from the liver passed through the great vein of the body, the vena cava, to the right side of the heart because of its dilative action, or diastole. Simultaneously, air, containing "vital spirits," acquired from the lungs was pulled from the venous artery into the left side of the heart. As the heart contracted, systole, blood was forced from the right side into the arterial vein for the nourishment of the lungs and also through the median septum into the left side of the heart. Since the thirteenth century, Arabian physicians had known that Galen's explanation of the passage of the blood through the septum was false. Columba's observation that the septum is too solid to permit the passage of blood and his conclusions that the blood enters the right side of the heart from the vena cava and leaves by the pulmonary artery, that it returns from the lungs by the pulmonary vein into the left side and leaves through the aorta, comes close to Harvey's eventual discovery of the circulation of the blood.

Mention also must be made of another precursor of Harvey: Catalan-born Michael Servetus (1511–53). Better known because of his unitarian views of the Godhead, he suffered the unique fate of being executed for heresy by both the Catholics and Protestants. He was burned in effigy by the Inquisition in Lyons in June 1553 and met his fate at the stake in Geneva in October of the same year. Servetus' interpretation of the circulation of the blood, published in 1533, is almost identical with that of Columba:

Communication between the two ventricles does not take place in the center of the heart as is generally believed, but by means of the greatest artery through the right ventricle after it has pumped the purified blood through towards its long trip to the lungs. In the lungs it is transformed and turns red. From the vena arteriosa it flows into the arteria venosa where it combines with the air inhaled to such an extent that it is able to shed its impurities by means of exhalation. Finally it flows into the left side of the heart as a result of dilation where it becomes life spirit.

None of Harvey's precursors, however, recognized the systemic circulation nor were they able to explain circulation on a quantitative and experimental basis.

Harvey returned to England in 1602 and, after private practice in London, was appointed lecturer to the College of Physicians in 1615. From his lecture notes, it is apparent that his theories were already moving away from the Galenic position. It is not quite certain when he arrived at his great discovery, probably in 1635. We know that he spent a great deal of time, from 1616 onward, in dissecting animals such as dogs, fish, frogs, and eels. His epoch-making book, the *Exercitatio Anatomica de Motu Cordis et Sanguinis in Animalibus,* appeared in Frankfurt in 1628. It is regarded as a landmark in medical history, as it did not merely theorize that the blood circulated—it proved it by morphological, mathematical, and experimental arguments.

The following selections sum up in Harvey's own words the essence of his discovery:

In connection with the motions of the heart these things are further to be observed having reference to the motions and pulses of the arteries.

1. At the moment the heart contracts, and when the breast is struck, when in short the organ is in its state of systole, the arteries are dilated, yield a pulse, and are in a state of diastole. In like manner, when the right ventricle contracts and propels its charge of blood, the pulmonary artery is distended at the same time with the other arteries of the body.

2. When the left ventricle ceases to act, to contract, to pulsate, the pulse in the arteries also ceases; further, when this ventricle contracts languidly, the pulse in the arteries is scarcely perceptible. In like manner, the pulse in the right ventricle failing, the pulse in the pulmonary artery ceases also.

3. Further, when an artery is divided or punctured, the blood is seen to be forcibly propelled from the wound the moment the left ventricle contracts; and, again, when the pulmonary artery is wounded, the blood will be

seen spouting forth with violence at the instant when the right ventricle contracts.

So also in fishes, if the vessel which leads from the heart to the gills be divided, at the moment when the heart becomes tense and contracted, at the same moment does the blood flow with force from the divided vessel.

In the same way, when we see the blood in arteriotomy projected now to a greater, now to a less distance, and that the greater jet corresponds to the diastole of the artery and to the time when the heart contracts and strikes the ribs, and is in a state of systole, we understand that the blood is expelled by the same movement.

From these facts it is manifest, in opposition to commonly received opinions, that the diastole of the arteries corresponds with the time of the heart's systole; and that the arteries are filled and distended by the blood forced into them by the contraction of the ventricles; the arteries, therefore, are distended, because they expand like bellows. It is in virtue of one and the same cause, therefore, that all the arteries of the body pulsate, viz., the contraction of the left ventricle; in the same way as the pulmonary artery pulsates by the contraction of the right ventricle.

Finally, that the pulses of the arteries are due to the impulses of the blood from the left ventricle, may be illustrated by blowing into a glove, when the whole of the fingers will be found to become distended at one and the same time, and in their tension to bear some resemblance to the pulse. For in the ratio of the tension is the pulse of the heart, fuller, stronger, and more frequent as that acts more vigorously, still preserving the rhythm and volume, and order of the heart's contractions. Nor is it to be expected that because of the motion of the blood, the time at which the contraction of the heart takes place, and that at which the pulse in an artery (especially a distant one) is felt, shall be otherwise than simultaneous: it is here the same as in blowing up a glove or bladder; for in a plenum (as in a drum, a long piece of timber, etc.) the stroke and the motion occur at both extremities at the same time. Aristotle, too, has said, "the blood of all animals palpitates within their veins (meaning the arteries), and by the pulse is sent everywhere simultaneously." And further, "thus do all the veins pulsate together and by successive strokes, because they all depend upon the heart; and, as it is always in motion, so are they likewise always moving together, but by successive movements." It is well to observe with Galen, in this place, that the old philosophers called the arteries veins.

* * *

And now I may be allowed to give in brief my view of the circulation of the blood, and to propose it for general adoption.

Since all things, both argument and ocular demonstration, show that the blood passes through the lungs, and heart by the force of the ventricles, and is sent for distribution to all parts of the body, where it makes its way into the veins and porosities of the flesh, and then flows by the veins from the circumference on every side to the centre, from the lesser to the greater veins, and is by them finally discharged into the vena cava and the right auricle of the heart, and this in such a quantity or in such a flux and reflux thither by the arteries, hither by the veins, as cannot possibly be supplied by the ingesta, and is much greater than can be required for mere purposes of nutrition; it is absolutely necessary to conclude that the blood in the animal body is impelled in a circle, and is in a state of ceaseless motion; that this is the act or function which the heart performs by means of its pulse; and that it is the sole and only end of the motion and contraction of the heart. (*De Motu Cordis,* Cap. III)

Like Vesalius before him, Harvey encountered widespread resistance. And not all his critics were physicians. Churchmen were reluctant to accept the heart, so prominent in biblical language, as a mere muscular pump. Even after more than three centuries, literature still alludes to the heart as the center of emotions. In 1654, Harvey was elected president of the College of Physicians. A strong monarchist, he had remained loyal to Charles I, whose friend and physician he was during the Civil War.

Thomas Hobbes (1588–1679), who heralded in England the new era of the Enlightenment, was deeply influenced by Harvey. In the preface to his *Elements of Philosophy,* he refers to Harvey as the founder of scientific physiology because it was developed in terms of motion. Harvey, he remarks with envy, was the only man he knew who was able to conquer prejudice sufficiently to achieve the complete revolution of a science within his lifetime. It is to the Enlightenment that we must now turn to see the fruition of the Renaissance innovations.

6

The Age of the Enlightenment

THE GERMAN philosopher Immanuel Kant gave an enduring description of the Enlightenment when he referred to it as the liberation of the autonomous human being who is capable of using his mind without the tutelage of others. Its slogan he terms *"sapere aude"* (dare to know). For sheer audacity in learning, no other era has surpassed the seventeenth and eighteenth centuries. In recent years, historians have come to speak not only of an Enlightenment but of a *Frühaufklärung,* or pre-Enlightenment, so that although the movement is still identified with the era of Locke and Voltaire its general characteristics are already evident in the early seventeenth century. The changed attitude toward the role of science and the decline of theology are already discernible at this early period. Religion, which had played such a dominant role in the preceding age, was gradually replaced by a belief in science and reason. The idea of human progress replaced the traditional belief in a fallen mankind doomed to sorrow and misery. There was, in the words of H. Butterfield, "a colossal secularization of thought." Materialism and atheism were often taught and defended. Physician Julien Offray de la Mettrie (1709–51) is perhaps the extreme example of this materialistic rationalism. In his *L'homme machine,* he taught that everything spiritual was a delusion and that man will never be truly happy until theologians have abandoned their squabbles and nature has asserted her claims.

The disassociation of religion and life is probably best typified in the realm of art. In contrast to the Renaissance, when a religious motif was paramount in the work of all the major painters, sculptors, and architects, during the Enlightenment there was no example of such

103

exclusiveness. Society during this period was not only secularized; it became more cosmopolitan and more mobile both physically and socially. Politically, the Peace Treaty of Westphalia (1648), which had finally terminated the religious wars resulting from the Reformation, set the national boundaries of Europe until the time of the French Revolution. Culturally, the seventeenth and eighteenth centuries were dominated by the Baroque. In painting, architecture, music, and literature, there was a new element of individualism: a new clarity, energy, and emotional appeal. A passion for technology permeated every aspect of life. Armed with mathematically controlled technology, man began not only to assess and study nature but to conquer it. It is from the Enlightenment that many of the characteristics of the twentieth century have derived: a vogue for science, humanitarianism, the basic concepts of democracy, and the statistical method of studying social phenomena.

No understanding of the Enlightenment is possible without a knowledge of the man whose ideas dominated it: René Descartes (1596–1650). He was born at Le Haye in Touraine and received his early education at the Jesuit College of Henry IV in Le Fleche. The curriculum there was traditionally Aristotelian, and the brilliant student was well grounded in the philosophical system that he was later to do so much to undermine. After receiving a license in law from the University of Poitier, where he also studied anatomy, he joined the armies of Maurice of Nassau, and after a few years of soldiering, he settled down in the Netherlands, where he devoted himself to the study of mathematics, physics, optics, and medicine, with the hope of creating a "universal science."

It was Descartes's aim to bring about a single-handed reconstruction of philosophy by revolutionizing the very notion of philosophy itself. His approach of universal doubt, *de omnibus dubitandum est,* became the slogan of educated Europeans for the next two centuries.

In order to close the gap between science and wisdom, he emphasized that wisdom is a matter of scientific reason rather than of erudition. Philosophical wisdom as based on the natural use of reason does not need to rely on revelation and theology. It is the work of man as man and is oriented toward man's welfare and permanent happiness. The mysteries of nature and the laws of mathematics could both be unlocked by the same key. The essence of material substances is an extension from which proceed divisibility, figurability, and mobility.

For Descartes, the body is a machine that operates by an impulse received from the soul, which he locates in the pineal gland. There are but two physiological principles: motion and warmth. God, he explains, has placed in the hearts of man and animals a vital warmth that promotes the circulation of the blood and separates from the blood its finest and most noble particles, which constitute the animal spirits. This fluid carries the stimulation of the senses to the pineal gland and, returning through the nerves to the muscles, carries the impulse of motion from the pineal gland to the limbs. Thus, in contrast to the traditional dualism of Aristotle, soul and matter, he substitutes mind and body. By establishing a more anthropocentric philosophy, Descartes exerted a profound influence on the study of medicine. Early in his career, he declared that if any great improvement in the condition of mankind was to be achieved medicine would provide the means. His *De Homine,* written in 1622 and published after his death, is regarded as the first European textbook on physiology. His *Discours de la méthode,* published in 1637, exerted the greatest influence on contemporary Europe. Here he explains the notion of the body as a machine:

But there are many other circumstances which prove that what I have alleged is the true cause of the motion of the blood. In the first place, the difference that is observed between the blood which flows from the veins, and that from the arteries, can only arise from this, that being rarefied, and, as it were, distilled by passing through the heart, it is thinner, and more vivid, and warmer immediately after leaving the heart, in other words, when in the arteries, than it was a short time before passing into either, in other words, when it was in the veins; and if attention be given, it will be found that this difference is very marked only in the neighbourhood of the heart; and is not so evident in parts more remote from it. In the next place, the consistency of the coats of which the arterial vein and the great artery are composed, sufficiently shows that the blood is impelled against them with more force than against the veins. And why should the left cavity of the heart and the great artery be wider and larger than the right cavity and the arterial vein, were it not that the blood of the venous artery, having only been in the lungs after it has passed through the heart, is thinner, and rarefies more readily, and in a higher degree, than the blood which proceeds immediately from the hollow vein? And what can physicians conjecture from feeling the pulse unless they know that according as the blood changes its nature it can be rarefied by the warmth of the heart, in a higher or lower degree, and more or less quickly than before? And if it be inquired how this heat is communicated to the other members, must it not be admitted that this is effected by means of the blood, which, passing through the heart, is there heated anew, and thence diffused over all the body? Whence it happens, that if the blood be withdrawn from any part, the heat is likewise withdrawn by the same means; and although the heart were as hot as glowing iron, it would not be capable of warming the feet and hands as at present, unless it continually sent thither new blood. We likewise perceive from this, that the true use of respiration is to bring sufficient fresh air into the lungs, to cause the blood which flows into them from the right ventricle of the heart, where it has been rarefied and, as it were, changed into vapours, to become thick, and to convert it anew into blood, before it flows into the left cavity, without which process it would be unfit for the nourishment of the fire that is there. This receives confirmation from the circumstance, that it is observed of animals destitute of lungs that they have also but one cavity in the heart, and that in children who cannot use them while in the womb, there is a hole through which the blood flows from the hollow vein into the left cavity of the heart, and a tube through which it passes from the arterial vein into the grand artery without passing through the lung.

In the next place, how could digestion be carried on in the stomach unless the heart communicated heat to it through the arteries, and along with this certain of the more fluid parts of the blood, which assist in the dissolution of the food that has been taken in? Is not also the operation which converts the juice of food into blood easily comprehended, when it is considered that it is distilled by passing and repassing through the heart perhaps more than one or two hundred times in a day? And what more need be adduced to explain nutrition, and the production of the different humours of the body, beyond saying, that the force with which the blood, in being rarefied, passes from the heart towards the extremities of the arteries, causes certain of its parts to remain in the members at which they arrive, and there occupy the place of some others expelled by them; and that according to the situation, shape, or smallness of the pores with which they meet, some rather than others flow into certain parts, in the same way that some sieves are observed to act, which, by being variously perforated, serve to separate different species of grain? And, in the last place, what above all is here worthy of observation, is the generation of the animal spirits, which are like a very subtle wind, or rather a very pure and vivid flame which, continually ascending in great abundance from the heart to the brain, thence penetrates through the nerves into the muscles, and gives motion to all the members; so that to account for other parts of the blood which, as most agitated and penetrating, are the fittest to compose these spirits, proceeding towards the brain, it is not necessary to suppose any other cause, than simply, that the arteries which carry them thither proceed from the heart in the most direct lines, and that, according to the rules of mechanics, which are the same with those of nature, when many objects tend at once to the same point where there is not sufficient room for all (as is the case with the parts of the blood which flow forth from the left cavity of the heart and tend towards the brain), the weaker and less agitated parts must necessarily be driven aside from that point by the stronger which alone in this way reach it.

I had expounded all these matters with sufficient minuteness in the treatise which I formerly thought of publishing. And after these, I had shown what must be the fabric of the nerves and muscles of the human body to give the animal spirits contained in it the power to move the members, as when we see heads shortly after they have been struck off still move and bite the earth, although no longer animated; what changes must take place in the brain to produce waking, sleep, and dreams; how light, sounds, odours, tastes, heat, and all the other qualities of external objects impress it with different ideas by means of the senses; how hunger, thirst, and other internal affections can likewise impress upon it divers ideas; what must be understood by the common sense in which these ideas are received, by the memory which retains them, by the fantasy which can change them in various ways, and out of them compose new ideas, which, by the same means, distributing the animal spirits through the muscles, can cause the members of such a body to move in as many different ways, and in a manner as suited, whether to the objects that are presented to its senses or to its internal affections, as can take place in our own case apart from the guidance of the will. Nor will this appear at all strange to those who are acquainted with the variety of movements performed by the different automata, or moving machines fabricated by human industry, and that with help of but few pieces compared with the great multitude of bones, muscles, nerves, arteries, veins, and other parts that are found in the body of each animal. Such persons will look upon this body as a machine made by the hands of God which is incomparably better arranged, and adequate to movements more admirable than is any machine of human invention. (*Discours de la Méthode,* V)

In contrast to the Middle Ages and the Renaissance, when the body was considered a work of art and the teleological aspects of its functions emphasized, the scientists of the Enlightenment came to regard the body as a machine. As such, it was subject to the newly discovered laws of nature. Two schools of thought evolved: the iatrophysical and the iatrochemical. The former, influenced by Descartes, held that all physiological phenomena should be treated according to the rigid laws of physics; the latter, influenced by Jean van Helmont (1577–

1644), a student of Paracelsus, taught that all corporeal activity was purely chemical. Although neither school produced any lasting effect on medicine, largely because of the inadequacies of both physics and chemistry at that time, both systems did pave the way for the more genuine scientific progress of modern times. In a certain sense, moreover, many of the problems they posed remain unanswered to this day.

Descartes's concern with medicine was but one aspect of a wideranging interest in scientific subjects. He was the first to introduce exponents, thereby laying the groundwork for calculus and analytical geometry. His experiments in optics led to the discovery of the law of refraction, and his research with lenses, whereby light rays were converged at a point, marks him as a pioneer in the field of microscopy. Discovered, apparently by accident, by the Dutch spectaclemakers Johannes Jansen and his son Zacharias at the end of the sixteenth century, the microscope was popularized largely through the work of Galileo. Although Jan Swammerdam (1637–80) and Athanasius Kircher (1602–80) had both used this new invention, it was the Dutch-born Anton van Leeuwenhoek (1632–1723) whose studies had the greatest impact on medical history. He was the first to see protozoa under the microscope and to give accurate descriptions of bacterial clumps as well as individual spirilla and bacilli. In describing spermatozoa, red blood corpuscles, and the striped character of voluntary muscle, he demonstrated that the method of free inquiry advocated by Descartes could lead even the untrained to high achievement.

Leeuwenhoek's renown was due to the fact that, although uneducated, he managed to have his discoveries achieve international fame by submitting them to scientific societies in England and France. A distinguishing feature of the Enlightenment was that the natural sciences were no longer the domain of isolated, although brilliant, men of genius. There was a dramatic shift from science as an individual enterprise to science as an institutionalized activity. This phenomenon can be explained in part by the conservatism of the traditional strongholds of organized learning, the universities, and in part by the fact that governments began to realize the beneficial uses of the new science. The peculiar economic and social conditions of the seventeenth and eighteenth centuries made it possible for a large number of self-educated and otherwise unemployed gentlemen to devote themselves to scientific investigation and to present their findings to organized groups. Associations, or academies as they were called, formed with the express purpose of furthering scientific knowledge, appeared in most of the nations of western Europe during this period.

One of the earliest of the academies of science was the Accademia dei Lincei, founded in Rome in 1601. Galileo, whose experiments led to the introduction of the pulsilogium, or pulse clock, and the spirit thermometer, was a member of this group. In 1662, the Royal Society of London for the Promotion of Natural Knowledge was chartered in England. The Académie Royale des Sciences was established in France in 1666 by Colbert. In Germany, although there were no scientific academies until the eighteenth century, there were active scientific groups, such as the Collegium Naturae Curiosorum, founded in 1652 by Lorentz Bausch. There was a considerable exchange of ideas between the various associations, and all of them published their findings in scholarly journals. In France, the Académie published the *Journal des Savants,* and in England, *The Philosophical Transactions of the Royal Society,* published monthly, became the chief vehicle of the new learning. During his lifetime, Leeuwenhoek sent more than four hundred scientific papers to both the Royal Society and the Académie. The discovery of the capillary anastomosis between the arteries and the veins, completing Harvey's explanation of blood circulation, although discovered by the Italian Marcello Malphigi (1628–94), was given wider credence through the papers of Leeuwenhoek.

Malphigi is regarded as one of the most versatile and accomplished scientists of his time. He obtained his medical degree at the University of Bologna in 1653 and was appointed to a chair at the university, where he worked with Giovanni Borelli, proponent of the Iatrophysical school of medicine. He later taught at Bologna and Messina and for the final years of his life was personal physician to Pope Innocent XII. In addition to his discovery of the capillaries between the arteries and the veins, Malphigi is considered the founder of descriptive embryology by reason of his work *De Formatione pulli in Ovo,* published in 1673. He also described the sensory papillae and taste buds and made microscopic analyses of the skin, spleen, liver, and kidney. In his *De Recentorum medicorum studio,* he proposed changes in medical curricula based upon experimental philosophy and reason that antedate what is today termed basic research.

As in the previous century, Italian scientists continued to dominate the field of medical studies. Francesco Redi (1626–94) pioneered in the field of bacteriology by attacking the notion of spontaneous generation. Gasparo Aselli (1581–1626), professor of surgery at Pavia, explored the mysteries of digestion, discovering the lacteals of the mesentery in dogs, thus leading to the later discoveries of the lymphatic system. Giovanni Borelli (1608–79) furthered the work of Harvey by explaining the role of the nerves in heart action and by proving that the heart's temperature was the same as the rest of the body, thus putting to rest the erroneous belief that the heart was the source of bodily warmth. His *De Motu Animalium,* published in 1679, set forth in clear terms the mechanics of muscular action. Bernardino Ramazzini (1633–1714), who taught at the universities of Modena and Padua, is of special interest because of his work *De Moribus Artificium,* a study of occupational diseases. In it, he describes the ailments of some fifty-two different professions and occupations. Translated into English, Dutch, and French, the work has been described as the first history of industrial medicine and hygiene because it fostered social aspects of preventive medicine.

Giovanni Lancisi (1654–1720), personal physician to three popes, reflects the continuing versatility of his generation of scientist-practitioners. He was distinguished as an anatomist, botanist, and epidemiologist. In his work *De noxiis paludum effluvis,* published in 1717, he suggests that malaria may be caused by mosquitoes. His *De Motu Cordis et Aneurysmatibus* is considered a landmark in the history of cardiology. One of his most influential works was the *De Subitaneis Mortibus (On Sudden Deaths).* In the following passage, he describes the rupture of the vena cava:

HISTORY

Stephen Ascieri, a cobbler from the Januan quarter and past sixty, of corpulent build, and for eight years, around the time of the equinox, badly bothered with gout of the feet and of the hands (podagra and chiragra), started to become an invalid two years ago because of a cough coupled with a difficulty in breathing. From then on he suffered from palpitation of the heart and from some sort of hidden heaviness underneath the right side of the sternum, and experienced at times acute pain extending even to the shoulder, constriction of the chest, and heavy pulsation.

Very recently, during the course of the past winter, he was also rather frequently seized with vertigo accompanied by an appreciable calorification of the head and a sudden loss of strength. Because of this he became frequently disabled for cobbling. He got through half of the lenten season on pickled fish. Finally, on the 14th of March 1706, at 17 o'clock, when after luncheon he had guzzled down straight wine, he fell instantly dead from aphonia and angor.

THE DISSECTION OF THE BODY

It seemed to us, of course, like a marvel that not a single viscus contained in the abdomen should have deviated from the laws for their natural condition and position; in fact, the individual viscera turned out to be splendidly constituted in color, size and substance. The cystic bile alone showed something that was rather dark.

On the other hand, the thorax presented to us a frightful spectacle. For when the sternum was lifted (which in its right part was more elevated than in the left), the right lung, overly red and completely joined to the pleura, and looking as though a large hard body had grown onto it, excited our curiosity, so that we might all the more diligently clarify the novelty of this matter. For right beyond the pericardium lay hidden an aneurysm of the aorta. Then, when the knife was brought into play, we encountered immediately a bony lamella, oval in shape, which had taken hold of the external part of the dilated artery by means of which it adhered to the sternum and the ribs. Underneath that lamella and around the cavity of the first part of the ascending aorta, we found a polyplike substance, very similar to lard, incrusted with great neatness into an arch, such as it had never been granted to us elsewhere to discover its like in a large number of aneurysms. For indeed it was observed that this body appeared to have been previously melted by extreme heat and soon after solidified by extreme cold. In fact, it did not allow itself to be pulled apart into multiple laminas, like into so many sheets (as is everywhere usual). From this it is clear that a powerful obstruction against the pulsation of the blood toward the external parts had been erected. However, on that surface with which the lungs come in contact, we found the aorta blocked by and covered with a smaller polyplike barrier. Meanwhile the cavity of the aneurysm turned out to be so wide that it would readily have admitted a fist, and was so filled with grumelike blood, that it was evidently incapable of holding any further fluid. Nevertheless it was nowhere supplied with any sizeable opening, though we grant that at the base of the heart within the pericardium and at the lower side of the aneurysm, some certain dark striae, indications perhaps of larger, future apertures, had been observed. The length of this particular aneurysm did not exceed half the length of the aorta where this is curved, and this aorta in consequence preserved very nicely, both above as well as next to the heart, its natural diameter, and also, and this in excellent repair, the strength of its fibers.

But even here we had not reached the end of the evils. For indeed, as we were examining the pericardium, extremely swollen and nevertheless soft, we came to suspect some sort of a latent abnormal fluid. And of course, when cut, it yielded an immense quantity of blood, in fact as large an amount as it could possibly contain, which had been effused and turned into grume, and which, to be sure, exceeded two pounds in weight. This blood, indeed, had poured out, when within the vestibule of the vena cava next to the right auricle, a hole of about one inch in diameter had been opened. That this hole had been gradually made into the texture of this vestibule by an eroding liquid, was clearly shown by its edges, which were observed as not severed into shreds and lappets but just as though they had been thoroughly polished by a file. However, that the blood had not poured much sooner into the pericardium, was in all likelihood prevented by that delicate tunic with which the muscular covering ends, and which, as it extended above the hiatus, shut off any egress, and the tenuous fragments of this tunic were seen to be hanging as far as the extremities of the ulcer.

Finally, when the cranium had been cut, black blood flowed abundantly from the accidentally injured posterior sinus of the dura mater, and this type of blood was likewise contained in great quantity in the lateral sinuses. The ventricles of the brain were tumid with a clear serum which had overflown toward the start of the spinal medulla." (*De Subieaneis Mortibus,* Lib. II, Obs. 5)

The pathological and anatomical advances represented by Lancisi climaxed in the accomplishments of Giovani Batista Morgagni (1682–1771), professor at the University of Padua for almost half a century. To Morgagni belongs the honor of making pathology a genuine branch of modern science. The great German medical historian Rudolf Virchow claims that modern medicine begins with Morgagni. His five-column volume *De sedibus et causis morborum per anatonem indagatis* is considered one of the classics of medical literature. It is the first book in which autopsies are arranged and indexed in such a way as to present detailed histories, symptoms, and treatment in an ordered manner. The book was translated into English in 1769 by Benjamin Alexander and profoundly influenced medical study in England as well as in the colonies. The work examined an almost inexhaustible variety of ailments. The humoral concept in pathology was eradicated largely as a result of his studies. For Morgagni, the organ rather than the body became the ultimate unit in pathology. In a sense, he revolutionized medical methods of observation by uniting postmortem findings with clinical symptoms. His studies led to the eventual discovery of the sympathetic nervous system, the effect of alcoholism on the arteries, and the treatment of cancer by the surgical removal of malignant tumors.

The Italians may have been preeminent in medicine during the seventeenth century because of the excellence and multiplicity of their universities. Almost every principality had its own institution of higher learning, and patronage had a centuries-old tradition. In England, by contrast, only two institutions, Oxford and Cambridge, granted medical degrees. There was no medical university in London, where wonderful opportunities for clinical study could have been provided by the medieval foundations of St. Bartholomew, St. Thomas, and Bethlehem. The London Hospital College was not founded until 1786. It did not, however, grant medical degrees. Although France had a large number of medical faculties, some twenty under the old regime, most of them retained their medieval character until the French Revolution.

The outstanding name in English medicine during this period was Thomas Sydenham (1624–89). A member of Cromwell's army, he was educated at Oxford and was appointed as a Fellow of All Souls College, largely through political patronage. Political considerations also may account for the fact that he did not receive a license until 1663 nor a medical degree until four years later. After the Restoration, royalist London had little sympathy for Cromwellian supporters. Sydenham's Puritan convictions are reflected in his simple philosophy of medicine, which scoffed at theories and speculation. Throughout his life, he maintained an open hostility to the new developments in anatomy and physics, although he was on friendly terms with Robert Boyle.

His first published work, *Methodus Curandi Febres (A Method for Curing Fevers)*, published in 1666, shows that in many ways he was a traditionalist. His medical philosophy was basically Hippocratic: reliance on observation and common sense. Most contagion, he taught, was due to atmospheric or subterranean conditions. In 1683, he published his most important study, *Tractatus de podagra et hydrope,* a study of gout, from which he and so many of his compatriots suffered. Sydenham was one of the first to popularize the use of quinine in the treatment of fevers. The new medicament, a powder obtained from the bark of the cinchona, was introduced into Europe from Ecuador by the Jesuits in the 1630s. The fact that quinine cured without the usual evacuations demanded by the proponents of the humoral theory helped to undermine this vestige of ancient practice.

Sydenham's firsthand accounts of various diseases gave him an international reputation. In addition to gout and malarial fevers, he wrote detailed descriptions of measles, bronchopneumonia, scarlet fever, dysentery, and hysteria. Because of his great reliance upon the healing powers of nature and the wide spectrum of his knowledge of diseases, he has been referred to as the English Hippocrates, a title he has shared with a man born in the year of his death: Herman Boerhaave.

Boerhaave was born in the village of Voorhout, not far from the city of Leyden, the son of a Calvinist minister. Following the wishes of his father, he prepared himself for the ministry by combining the study of theology with that of medicine, a practice not uncommon among Mennonites and Quakers. In 1701, he was appointed a lector at the University of Leyden and eight years later was given the position of professor of medicine. From 1718 to 1729, he filled three chairs at the university: botany, chemistry, and medicine. The University of Leyden was founded in 1575 at the instigation of William the Silent, and by the early eighteenth century, it was one of the most important centers of learning in northern Europe. It is significant that its first faculty had been drawn from the University of Padua, and it continued to maintain the high standards of the latter's clinical schools. Boerhaave's predecessor there had been the famous Franciscus de le Boe Sylvius (1616–72), who was a chemist as well as an anatomist. His students, Graaf, Stensen, Swammerdam and van Horne, had given him an international reputation. Like Sylvius, Boerhaave was an extremely popular lecturer, attracting students from all parts of Europe. Between 1701 and 1738, more than two thousand medical students enrolled at Leyden, many of whom became important figures in the medical histories of their own countries: Van Swieten in Vienna, Hoffman in Germany, and Alexander Monro at Edinburgh. In addition, the Dutch physician published a number of textbooks that were translated from the Latin into French and English. His *Institutiones medicinae,* first published in 1708, went through fifteen Latin editions as well as a number of French and English translations. The *Aporismi de cognoscendis et curandis morbis* was published in England in 1733 under the title *Boerhaave's Aphorisms Concerning the Knowledge and Cure of Disease.* A synthesizer rather than a man of original thought, his writings have been compared to the medieval summas in their bringing together all extant medical knowledge. It was, above all, his method of bedside teaching that made Leyden a model for all of Europe. His student, Albrecht von Haller (1708–77), founder of medical bibliography, referred to him as the common teacher of Europe.

One of the most influential of Boerhaave's students was his secretary, Gerhard van Swieten (1700–72). The logical successor to the famous instructor of Leyden, he was passed over because of his Catholicism. He therefore accepted an invitation from the Empress Maria Teresa in 1745 to join her court in Vienna. He began as a lecturer at the court library and was later appointed to the medical faculty of the University of Vienna. Under his able direction, a "lying-in" clinic was established as a center for clinical instruction, and, it soon became one of the most important centers for medical study in Europe. A regulation that the hospitals of Vienna provide cadavers for postmortem examinations greatly advanced the development of pathological anatomy and the integration of practice and theory in medical instruction. Anton de Haen (1704–76), who succeeded van Swieten, is recalled because of his fifteen-volume work, *Ratio medendi,* one of the most comprehensive and detailed studies of clinical medicine to appear in that century.

Among the famous men of medicine associated with the early Vienna school were Leo Auenbrugger, Johann Frank, and Friedrich Mesmer. Auenbrugger was born at Gratz in lower Austria in 1722 and received his medical degree from the University of Vienna in 1752. After graduation, he accepted a position at the Spanish Military Hospital of the Holy Trinity, whose wards were used by the clinical department of the university for case demonstration. Ten years of experience resulted in the publication of his famous *Inventum Novum.* Auenbrugger recognized that diseases of the chest can be distinguished from one another and differentiated by the sound elicited when the chest is tapped with the finger:

THIRD OBSERVATION
Of the Preternatural or Morbid Sound of the Chest and Its General Import

To be able justly to appreciate the value of the various sounds elicited from the chest in cases of disease it is necessary to have learned, by experience on many subjects, the modifications of sound, general or partial, produced by the habit of the body, natural confirmation as to the scapulae, mammae, the heart, the capacity of the thorax, the degree of fleshiness, fatness, etc., etc.;

inasmuch as these various circumstances modify the sound considerably.

If, then, a distinct sound, equal on both sides, and commensurate to the degree of percussion, is not obtained from the sonorous regions above mentioned, a morbid condition of some of the parts within the chest is indicated.

On this truth a general rule is founded, and from this certain predictions can be deduced, as will be shown in order. For I have learned from much experience that diseases of the worst description may exist within the chest unmarked by any symptoms, and undiscoverable by any other means than percussion alone.

A clear and equal sound elicited from both sides of the chest indicates that the air cells of the lungs are free, and uncompressed either by a solid or liquid body. (Exceptions to this rule will be mentioned in their place.)

If a sonorous part of the chest struck with the same intensity yields a sound duller than natural, disease exists in that part.

If a sonorous region of the chest appears, on percussion, entirely destitute of the natural sound,—that is, if it yields only a sound like that of a fleshy limb when struck,—disease exists in that region.

The nature of the indications above pointed out will be understood by any one who attends to the difference of sound elicited by percussion of the chest and of the thigh in his own person.

The superficial extent of this unnatural sound in a sonorous region is commensurate with the extent of the morbid affection.

If a place naturally sonorous, and now sounding only as a piece of flesh when struck, still retains the same sound (on percussion) when the breath is held after a deep inspiration, we are to conclude that the disease extends deep into the cavity of the chest. If the same results are obtained both before and behind on points precisely opposite, we are to conclude that the disease occupies the whole diameter of the chest.

These varying results depend on the greater or less diminution of the volume of air usually contained in the thorax (lungs); and the cause which occasions this diminution, whether solid or liquid, produces analogous results to those obtained by striking a cask, for example, in different degrees of emptiness or fulness: the diminution of sound being proportioned to the diminution of the volume of air contained in it.

Johann Frank, who after 1795, was professor of clinical medicine at the University of Vienna, represents medicine as envisioned by the enlightened despot. A staunch supporter of the Emperor Joseph II's social reforms, he looked upon the health of the citizenry as a matter of public concern and state control. To this end, he spent most of his professional career in the writing of a multi-volume work entitled *Medicinische Polizie,* a complete system of medical policy. The first volume appeared in 1779 and the sixth and final volume in 1818, three years before his death. The work contains detailed discussions and recommendations on such matters as marital hygiene, child welfare, food inspection, and general sanitation. In short, it treats public health from the womb to the tomb. Many of Frank's suggestions appeared radical even in the enlightened Austria of Joseph II. For example, he recommended that unmarried mothers and their children be cared for out of state funds. His proposals that those who were mentally and physically fit should marry and that celibacy was an unhealthy state did not endear him to the clergy of Catholic Austria. Yet many of his ideas have been incorporated into the laws of the Western world.

Friedrich Mesmer (1734–1815), while not directly associated with the Vienna school, attained notoriety in the Austrian capital because of his alleged cures through hypnotism. A number of quasi-miraculous cures that he effected by means of animal magnetism forced him to move to Paris, where he soon attracted a large following, the *Société de l'harmonie.* Among his many disciples was Lafayette, who attempted to induct George Washington into the mysteries of Mesmerism.

Another maverick of the Austrian school, who, like Mesmer, found refuge in Paris, was Franz Joseph Gall (1758–1828). A student of van Swieten, Gall is considered the father of phrenology because he attempted to localize mental functions and diseases by studying the cranium from the outside. During the early nineteenth century, the school of Vienna regained some of its international fame through the work of Josef Skoda (1805–81) and Karl Rokitansky (1804–78). Skoda distinguished himself by improving the methods of percussion and auscultation discovered by Auenbrugger and popularized by Laenec. Rokitansky gained international fame because of his work in pathological anatomy. He was the first to discover the difference between lobar- and bronchopneumonia and to describe the microscopic appearance of emphysema. During the nineteenth century, the Vienna school of medicine, because of its method of scientific bedside teaching, became the leading medical school of all Europe. It was particularly attractive to American students who wanted to specialize, and some twenty-one thousand studied there. An American Medical Association of Vienna, which exists to this day, was founded in 1904.

The University of Edinburgh also came under the influence of Boerhaave, five of whose students are regarded as the founding fathers of the medical school there. Although the university had been established in 1583, it did not possess a medical school until 1726. In 1720, after completing his studies at Leyden, Alexander Monro (1697–1767), whose father, of the same name, was a surgeon in the army of William of Orange, was appointed to a chair of anatomy. This marked the beginning of a trend in excellence that was to make Edinburgh one of the greatest schools of medicine in the West, certainly in the British Isles. Like the University of Vienna, the Edinburgh school utilized the clinical facilities of local hospitals, especially the Royal Infirmary, to combine theory and practice. By the end of the century, the Scottish university was supplying a larger number of professionally trained physicians than any other school in the British Isles. The co-founders of North America's first medical school at the University of Pennsylvania, William Shipper (1738–1808) and John Morgan (1735–89), were both graduates of Edinburgh. A look at some of the more distinguished practitioners associated with this institution offers a good basis for its claim to greatness.

William Cullen (1712–90) founded a system based on the theory that the muscle was a continuation of the nerve and that life itself was simply a matter of nervous energy. In a work published in 1769, *Synopsis nosologiae methodicae,* he followed the classification system of Swedish botanist Linnaeus by arranging all diseases according to orders, genera, and species. His *First Lines on the Practice of Physics* became a handbook for practitioners in England as well as in the colonies. Cullen's theories were later attacked by one of his own students, the ill-fated John Brown (1735–88). Brown, who died as a result of overdosage of drugs and alcoholism, fathered a system known as Brunonism. The system was eclectic, with borrowings from the ancient Methodists and the theories of Boerhaave's student Albrecht von Haller. Haller had earlier discovered that irritability is a specific property of all muscle tissue and that sensibility is the exclusive property of nervous tissue. Brown expanded this theory to claim that all life depended upon excitability. The "stimuli" on which life depends are either external or internal, local or universal. Health depends upon a well-balanced state of excitability. Hence, diseases were classified as either "sthenic," increased excitability, or "asthenic," decreased excitability. The latter were cured by stimulants, the former by sedatives. Brunonism was popular not only in England but in the colonies, France, and Germany. Robert Whytt (1714–66), also of Edinburgh, is noted for his work on the pathology of the nervous system, especially his demonstration that reflex actions are not dependent on the integrity of the spinal cord. In *Observations on the Dropsy in the Brain,* he described for the first time tubercular meningitis in children. John Pringle (1707–82), who was surgeon-general of the English army from 1743 until 1758, contributed to the advance of medicine with his publication of *Observations on the Diseases of the Army* in 1752. Here he focused attention on the need for better hygienic practices in military hospitals by urging better ventilation. Pringle's efforts to improve medical practices in the military were furthered by James Lind (1716–94), who received his medical degree from Edinburgh in 1748. His *Treatise on Scurvey,* published in 1753, was the result of nine years' experience as a naval surgeon with the British fleet. In spite of the Dutch success in eliminating this scourge by using sauerkraut and citrus fruits, the English were reluctant to accept this method. As late as the 1740s, the English circumnavigator of the globe, Admiral Anson, lost four-fifths of his crew from scurvy. Lind, by a series of experiments, proved that citrus fruit not only cured the disease but also prevented it. The English Navy began to provide its crewmen with a daily ration of citrus fruit, a practice that gave birth to the expression "limey."

William Withering (1741–99) was one of Edinburgh's noted botanists. His *Account of the Foxglove and Some of Its Medical Uses* is an important study on the use of digitalis in the treatment of cardiac diseases. The Hunter brothers, William and John, also made considerable contributions to British medicine during this period. William, who studied under Alexander Monro at Edinburgh, distinguished himself as an anatomist. His *Anatomy of the Gravid Uterus,* published in 1774, marks him as an English Vesalius. John, who, after many years as a surgeon at St. George's Hospital in London, was appointed Surgeon-General of the Army, wrote extensively on a variety of subjects. Among his works were *A Treatise on the Venereal Disease,* published in 1786, and *The Natural History of the Human Teeth,* the first scientific treatment of the teeth to appear in English. Perhaps the best-known physician in England during the Enlightenment was John Hunter's student Edward Jenner (1749–1823).

Jenner was born in Berkeley, the son of an Anglican vicar, and was apprenticed to John Hunter at the age of twenty-one. His teacher's great stress on experimentation led eventually to Jenner's discovery of preventive inoculation against smallpox. It is difficult to imagine what a terrible scourge smallpox was until comparatively recent times. It is estimated that one-tenth of all deaths in the eighteenth century were attributed to it, as were most cases of blindness. Smallpox had been treated for centuries in China by a process known as variolation, and this method had been introduced into Europe from Turkey in the early part of the century. However, its success had been sporadic and unscientific. It was the great achievement of Jenner that he placed inoculation on a scientific basis and dispelled the fear and repugnance of this method. In 1798, he published his famous *Inquiry into the Causes and Effects of the Variolae Vaccinae:*

The deviation of man from the stage in which he was originally placed by nature seems to have proved to him a prolific source of diseases. From the love of splendour, from the indulgences of luxury, and from his fondness for amusement he has familiarised himself with a great number of animals, which may not originally have been intended for his associates.

The wolf, disarmed of ferocity, is now pillowed in the lady's lap. The cat, the little tiger of our island, whose natural home is the forest, is equally domesticated and caressed. The cow, the hog, the sheep, and the horse, are all, for a variety of purposes, brought under his care and dominion.

There is a disease to which the horse, from his state of domestication, is frequently subject. The farriers have called it the grease. It is an inflammation and swelling in the heel, from which issues matter possessing properties of a very peculiar kind, which seems capable of generating disease in the human body (after it has undergone the modification which I shall presently speak of), which bears so strong a resemblance to the smallpox that I think it highly probable it may be the source of the disease.

In this dairy country a great number of cows are kept, and the office of milking is performed indiscriminately by men and maid servants. One of the former having been appointed to apply dressings to the heels of a horse affected with the grease, and not paying due attention to cleanliness, incautiously bears his part in milking the cows, with some particles of the infectious matter adhering to his fingers. When this is the case, it commonly happens that a disease is communicated to the cows, and from the cows to the dairy-maids, which spreads through the farm until the most of the cattle and domestics feel its unpleasant consequences. This disease has obtained the name of the cow-pox. It appears on the nipples of the cows in the form of irregular pustules. At their first appearance they are commonly of a palish blue, or rather of a colour somewhat approaching to livid, and are surrounded by an erysipelatous inflammation. These pustules, unless a timely remedy be applied, frequently degenerate into phagedenic ulcers, which prove extremely troublesome. The animals become indisposed, and the secretion of milk is much lessened. Inflamed spots now begin to appear on different parts of the hands of the domestics employed in milking, and sometimes on the wrists, which quickly run on to suppuration, first assuming the appearance of the small vesications produced by a burn. Most commonly they appear about the joints of the fingers and at their extremities; but whatever parts are affected, if the situation will admit, these superficial suppurations put on a circular form, with their edges more elevated than their centre, and of a colour distantly approaching to blue. Absorption takes place, and tumours appear in each axilla. The system becomes affected—the pulse is quickened; and shiverings, succeeded by heat, with general lassitude and pains about the loins and limbs, with vomiting, come on. The head is painful, and the patient is now and then even affected with delirium. These symptoms, varying in their degrees of violence, generally continue from one day to three or four, leaving ulcerated sores about the hands, which, from the sensibility of the parts, are very troublesome, and commonly heal slowly, frequently becoming phagendenic, like those from whence they sprung. The lips, nostrils, eyelids, and other parts of the body are sometimes affected with sores; but these evidently arise from their being heedlessly rubbed or scratched with the patient's infected fingers. No eruptions on the skin have followed the decline of the feverish symptoms in any instance that has come under my inspection, one only excepted, and in this case a very few appeared on the arms: they were very minute, of a vivid red colour and soon died away without advancing to maturation; so that I cannot determine whether they had any connection with the preceding symptoms.

Thus the disease makes its progress from the horse to the nipple of the cow, and from the cow to the human subject.

Morbid matter of various kinds, when absorbed into the system, may produce effects in some degree similar; but what renders the cow-pox virus so extremely singular is that the person who has been thus affected is forever after secure from the infection of the smallpox; neither exposure to the variolous effluvia, nor the insertion of the matter into the skin, producing this distemper.

In support of so extraordinary a fact, I shall lay before my reader a great number of instances.

Case I.—Joseph Merret, now an under gardener to the Earl of Berkeley, lived as a servant with a farmer near this place in the year 1770, and occasionally assisted in milking his master's cows. Several horses belonging to the farm began to have sore heels, which Merret frequently attended. The cows soon became affected with the cow-pox, and soon after several sores appeared on his hands. Swellings and stiffness in each axilla followed, and he was so much indisposed for several days as to be incapable of pursuing his ordinary employment. Previously to the appearance of the distemper among the cows there was no fresh cow brought into the farm, nor any servant employed who was affected with the cow-pox.

In April, 1795, a general inoculation taking place here, Merret was inoculated with his family; so that a period of twenty-five years had elapsed from his having the cow-pox to this time. However, though the variolous matter was repeatedly inserted into his arm, I found it impracticable to infect him with it; an efflorescence only, taking on an erysipelatous look about the centre, appearing on the skin near the punctured parts. During the whole time that his family had the smallpox, one of whom had it very full, he remained in the house with them, but received no injury from exposure to the contagion.

It is necessary to observe that the utmost care was taken to ascertain, with the most scrupulous precision, that no one whose case is here adduced had gone through the smallpox previous to these attempts to produce that disease.

Had these experiments been conducted in a large city, or in a populous neighbourhood, some doubts might have been entertained; but here, where population is thin, and where such an event as a person's having had the smallpox is always faithfully recorded, no risk of inaccuracy in this particular can arise.

Case II.—Sarah Portlock, of this place, was infected with the cow-pox when a servant at a farmer's in the neighbourhood, twenty-seven years ago.

In the year 1792, conceiving herself, from the circumstance, secure from the infection of the smallpox, she nursed one of her own children who had accidentally caught the disease, but no indisposition ensued. During the time she remained in the infected room, variolous matter was inserted into both her arms, but without any further effect than in the preceding case.

Case III.—John Phillips, a tradesman of this town, had the cow-pox at so early a period as nine years of age. At the age of sixty-two I inoculated him, and was very careful in selecting matter in its most active state. It was taken from the arm of a boy just before the commencement of the eruptive fever, and instantly inserted. It very speedily produced a sting-like feel in the part. An efflorescence appeared, which on the fourth day was rather extensive, and some degree of pain and stiffness were felt about the shoulder: but on the fifth day these symptoms began to disappear, and in a day or two after went entirely off, without producing any effect on the system.

Case IV.—Mary Barge, of Woodford, in this parish, was inoculated with variolous matter in the year 1791. An efflorescence of a palish red colour soon appeared about the parts where the matter was inserted, and spread itself rather extensively, but died away in a few days without producing any variolous symptoms. She has since been repeatedly employed as a nurse to smallpox patients, without experiencing any ill consequences. This woman had the cow-pox when she lived in the service of a farmer in this parish thirty-one years before.

After describing nineteen additional cases, Jenner goes on:

Although I presume it may be unnecessary to produce further testimony in support of my assertion "that the cow-pox protects the human constitution from the infection of the smallpox," yet it affords me considerable satisfaction to say that Lord Somerville, the President of the Board of Agriculture, to whom this paper was shewn by Sir Joseph Banks, has found upon inquiry that the statements were confirmed by the concurring testimony of Mr. Dolland, a surgeon, who resides in a dairy country remote from this, in which these observations were made. With respect to the opinion adduced "that the source of the infection is a peculiar morbid matter arising in the horse," although I have not been able to prove it from actual experiments conducted immediately under my own eye, yet the evidence I have adduced appears sufficient to establish it.

One of the great medical achievements of the later Enlightenment was in the field of chemistry. Before the late eighteenth century, it had lagged behind physics because of a continuing belief that the visible world was composed of three elements: salt, sulphur, and mercury. In spite of Boyle's distinction between a chemical element and a chemical compound, chemists had failed to emancipate themselves from the misconceptions of natural philosophy. The mechanistic theory of explaining chemical change, popularized by Descartes, continued to dominate this branch of science. Thus tainted with the vestiges of medieval alchemy and lacking any standard technological terminology comparable to that of Newtonian physics, chemists were further handicapped by a lack of communication. Illustrative of this was the work of German physician George Stahl (1660–1744), who had developed a theory that all materials that burn contain a colorless, odorless, tasteless, weightless substance called phlogiston. The phlogiston theory dominated chemical thought through much of the eighteenth century until overthrown in 1777 by French chemist Antoine Lavoisier (1743–94).

Lavoisier's work culminated the experiments carried out independently by Black, Priestly, and Cavendish in England and by Sheele in Sweden. Joseph Black (1728–99), one of the first to use quantitative methods in chemistry, was born in France of Scottish parents and received a medical degree from the University of Edinburgh in 1754. His thesis, a study of "magnesia alba," led to the realization that a certain gas that he called "fixed air" was combined in the alkalis and was different from atmospheric air. He later deduced that it was this "fixed air" that caused suffocation in mines and was involved in vegetable fermentation. The gas is what we today call carbon dioxide. Joseph Priestly (1733–1804), a dissident Anglican minister who later emigrated to Pennsylvania and became one of the founders of the Unitarian movement, also worked with fixed air. Experimenting with the effects of acids on metals, he discovered in 1777 what he termed "nitrous air" or nitric oxide and "marine acid air" or hydrogen chloride. Later discoveries included ammonia, sulphur dioxide, and carbon monoxide. During this same period, Swedish pharmacist Karl Scheele (1742–86), in his attempts to explain the process of combustion, concluded that air is composed of two different gases: "fire air," or oxygen, and "vitiated air," or nitrogen. Scheele is regarded by many as being the founder of organic chemistry. Among his later discoveries were tannic, benzoic, and uric acids. His study of the chemical effects of light, particularly on chloride of silver, led to the discovery of photography. Henry Cavendish (1731–1810) helped solve the problem of combustion with his discovery of "inflammable air," or hydrogen. He obtained hydrogen by dissolving zinc in vitriolic acid. In 1781, by using an electric spark, he exploded a mixture of common air and "inflammable air" to produce a dew analyzed as pure water. The all-important mystery of combustion and the true notion of respiration was about to be solved. Lavoisier established that what his predecessors had called "dephlogisted air" and "fire air" were the purest part of air, "vital air," or oxygen. Lavoisier, completing Cavendish's experiments, proved that water is not a simple substance but rather a compound of two airs.

Lavoisier's discovery led to the realization that organic substances are composed for the most part of carbon and hydrogen and that respiration is in fact a form of combustion. Soon after he had solved the riddle of the composition of air, he collaborated with a number of other French scientists in establishing a uniform set of terms for chemical elements and compounds. In 1787, a work entitled *Méthode de Nomenclature Chimique* was published and established the standard vocabulary of chemistry used to this day. Physicians no longer speak of oil of tartar, flowers of zinc, or powder of agorath. While less poetic than the old nomenclature, the new chemistry possessed a vocabulary that was international and precise.

Ironically, the man who discovered the true nature of water was executed by a revolutionary council in 1794 for allegedly "watering the tobacco supplies" of the nation. The instrument of execution was the vertically guided blade invented by French physician J. I. Guillotin (1738–1814).

In spite of the many medical advances made during the Enlightenment, the ideal of Descartes that science would ultimately solve mankind's problems was not realized. With few exceptions, the great names in medicine were identified with elitist groups, royal families, scientific societies, or the military. Public health was for the most part ignored or neglected. A study made of the hospitals in London and Paris at the end of the seventeenth century by Sir William Petty estimates that more than a quarter of the patients died because of wretched conditions. For many, hospitalization was considered a prelude to death. In German cities, hospital conditions were so vile that physicians considered assignment there as equivalent to the death penalty. Recovery from surgery was rare.

Bleeding of patients continued to be a panacea. In a popular English work by William Buchan, entitled *Domestic Medicine* (1799), bleeding is recommended "at the beginning of all inflammatory fevers, pleurisies and peripneumonies—all topical inflammation as those of the intestine, womb, bladder, stomach, kidneys, throat, etc. as also in the asthma, sciatic pains, coughs, headaches, rheumatism, the apoplexy, epilepsy, and bloody flux. After falls, blows, bruises, or any violent hurt received either externally or internally, bleeding is necessary. But in all disorders proceeding from a relaxation of the solids, and an impoverished state of the blood, as dropsies, cacochymies, etc. bleeding is improper."

During this time, the pedantic formalism and incompetence of the medical profession was frequently the object of literary criticism. In France, Molière constantly directed his satirical pen against the pedants of the profession, authoring five plays on the subject, the most well known being *Le Malade Imaginaire.* The administration of medical enemas was so much in vogue in France that the enema syringe became in caricature the symbol of the medical profession. Louis XVIII received no less than 312 enemas within one year.

Few writers surpassed Jonathan Swift in vitriolic disdain for "enlightened" medicine, as the following selection from Part Four of *Gulliver's Travels* attests:

Their fundamental is that all diseases arise from repletion, from whence they conclude that a great evacuation of the body is necessary, either through the natural passage or upwards at the mouth. Their next business is from herbs, minerals, gums, oils, shells, salts, juices, seaweed, excrements, barks of trees, serpents, toads, frogs, spiders, dead men's flesh and bones, birds, beasts and fishes, to form a composition for smell and taste the most abominable, nauseous and detestable they can possible contrive, which the stomach immediately rejects with loathing; and this they call a vomit; or else from the same storehouse, with some other poisonous additions, they command us to take in at the orifice above or below (just as the physician then happens to be disposed) a medicine equally annoying and disgustful to the bowels; which relaxing the belly, drives down all before it, and this they call a purge or a clyster. For nature (as the physicians allege) having intended the superior-anterior orifice only for the intromission of solids and liquids, and the inferior posterior for ejection, these artists ingeniously considering that in all diseases nature is forced out of her seat, therefore to replace her in it the body must be treated in a manner directly contrary, by interchanging the use of each orifice, forcing solids and liquids in at the anus, and making evacuations at the mouth.

But besides real diseases we are subject to many that are only imaginary, for which the physicians have invented imaginary cures; these have their several names, and so have the drugs that are proper for them, and with these our female Yahoos are always infested.

7

Medicine in
Industrialized Society

TWO IMPORTANT revolutions profoundly affected the course of medical history during the nineteenth century; neither of them, industrial in England and political in France, was sudden or spectacular but both had consequences that have shaped much of what is considered modern civilization. The Industrial Revolution began in England in the last decade of the eighteenth century and within the next hundred years had spread throughout Europe and North America. Although England was less populous and wealthy than France, a number of factors account for the origin of the Industrial Revolution there. In the first place, England was ideally suited to the development of industry and trade because large deposits of coal and iron, made accessible by improved mining methods and an excellent system of inland transportation, were at hand. Improved methods of agriculture also released a large body of laborers no longer needed on the farms.

Financially, England was superior to France. Since the sixteenth century, she had, through a wise colonial policy, accumulated a vast store of capital and regulated it through a superior banking system. England also possessed the largest merchant fleet in the world, with more than five thousand ships and a hundred thousand seamen capable of carrying manufactured goods to the corners of the earth. Unlike the other nations of Western Europe, England was not troubled with political unrest. The revolution of the seventeenth century had placed the aristocratic and mercantile classes in control of a stable constitutional government. The main thrust of the first phase of the revolution was in the textile industry. New inventions—the Flying Shuttle of

John Kay followed by the Spinning Jenny and the Spinning Frame—finally led to the introduction of the power loom in 1789. Steam power was now wedded to improved methods for spinning and weaving cotton and wool. By the 1850s, the revolution had spread to Germany, France, and Belgium.

The Industrial Revolution brought to fruition the advances made in the natural sciences during the eighteenth century. New methods of turning iron into steel made transportation by rail and steamboat economical. By mid-century not only textile manufacture but other industries such as milling, brewing, and munitions, also had been mechanized in England, France, and Germany. As the population of the cities doubled and, in some cases, quadrupled, problems of hygiene and sanitation became acute. Living in damp, vermin-infested basements and alleys, thousands of workers succumbed to cholera, tuberculosis, and other diseases. In industrial cities like Manchester and Liverpool, toilet facilities were almost nonexistent. Excrement was often piled as high as fifteen feet in poor neighborhoods; sewage disposal was all but unknown; water supplies were generally polluted. A mid-nineteenth century writer described the smell from the Thames as being "so bad as to make it questionable as to whether Parliament could continue to sit." The large influx of laborers into the industrial cities of England created social and economic problems on a scale that was unprecedented.

It was against this background of a growing mortality rate that the government gradually realized that health was its concern. *Medicinische Polizie* of Johann Frank had been published in 1818, and he had unquestionably broken ground in advocating school hygiene, better sewage systems, clean water supplies, and the organization of hospitals as matters for the state. Yet in England, Parliament did not established the first Board of Health until 1848. The legislation was largely due to the untiring efforts of Sir Edwin Chadwick, whose report on the *Sanitary Conditions of the Laboring Classes of Great Britain* is considered a milestone in the drive toward public hygiene and preventive medicine. The work, which described the conditions prevailing in working-class dwellings and factories, eventually led to a series of laws that made public health a national concern.

Chadwick's work was furthered by William Far (1807–83), who, as editor of the *British Annals of Medicine,* introduced the use of vital statistics to regulate public health. By giving mathematical expression to the rise and fall of epidemic diseases, he laid the foundation for modern public health.

Max von Pettenkoffer (1818–1901) must also be listed among those who brought legislation to bear upon the unsanitary conditions spawned by industrial urbanization. As professor of pathological chemistry at the University of Munich, he spent a lifetime trying to combat cholera and typhoid, which he felt were caused by contaminated waters. As a result, most of the states of Germany adopted systems of medical government based on more scientific methods. Chairs of hygiene were established at German universities, and public health officers were subsidized.

By the end of the century, hygienic improvements, especially sewage disposal and clean water, had reduced the high mortality rate of typhoid and other waterborne diseases. It was not until 1878, largely due to the cholera epidemic of 1872–73, that a National Board of Health was created in the United States.

Overcrowding and unsanitary living conditions were not the only dark side of the Industrial Revolution. The monotony of doing the same work over long periods of time, coupled with the nervousness of keeping pace with the machine, had profound psychological effects. Alcoholism, insanity, and suicide were the handmaidens of the new proletariat. As one historian of the period remarks: "The animal machine—breakable in the best case, subject to a thousand sources of suffering—is chained to the iron machine which knows no suffering and no weariness."

Alcoholism was especially rampant in England. In London, the consumption of gin reached incredible proportions during the eighteenth century. It was, according to Henry Fielding, "the principal sustenance of a hundred thousand people in this metropolis." Drink had become the curse of the working classes.

In 1789, Quaker physician John Lettsom (1744–1815) wrote one of the first studies on the effects of alcoholism.

Treatment of the mentally ill in a more sane and rational manner was first introduced in post-revolutionary France. Philippe Pinel (1755–1826), who practiced in Paris during the revolution, is regarded as the first physician to devote himself to the study of mental diseases. His *Traite Medico-Philosophique sur l'alienation mentale ou la manie* (1801), is a milestone in the history of mental disease. A similar study by German Johann Reil (1759–1813) was published in 1803.

Pinel's student Jean Esquirol (1772–1840) introduced statistical medicine and the reform of mental institutions. His stress on the emotional and affective roots of mental illness marks him as one of the pioneers in the study of psychiatry. In Germany, Wilhelm Griesinger (1817–68), whose work *Pathology and Therapy of Psychic Disorders* appeared in 1845, instituted studies that were to culminate in the works of Richard von Krafft-Ebing, Sigmund Freud, and Carl Jung.

The French Revolution, with its ideas of individual liberty, popular sovereignty, and national patriotism, must still be regarded as one of the most important events in modern history. Both the liberalism and the democracy of the West, as well as the socialism of the East, find their roots in this movement. Its impact on medical history has often been overshadowed by its more immediate egalitarian transformation; yet the reform of medical education was also equally phenomenal. The famous report on the reform of medical education presented by physician and chemist Antoine François de Fourcroy to the revolutionary convention in November 1794 can be regarded as the beginning of a new era in medical history. Stating that what had up to that time been lacking in schools of medicine, i.e. the practice and art of observation at the patient's bedside, would henceforth become one of the main parts of learning, the report led to the creation of the Central School of Health in Paris. (Two years earlier, all faculties of theology, medicine, arts, and law had been repressed throughout the republic.) The reform of 1795 brought about a balance between theory and practice and enforced clinical hospital attendance. It also united under the same authority the teaching of medicine and surgery, conjoining the theoretical aspects of medicine with the practical experience in laboratories and hospitals. Schools of health also were set up in Montpellier and Strasbourg. All physicians educated under the old regime were required to submit to a new licensing examination.

In 1803, an equally important decree divided physicians into two categories: health officers and doctors of medicine and surgery. The purpose of the *officiat* was to provide, with little cost of time and money, a body of health auxilliaries to practice in rural areas. The preparation of the *officiat* required either three years in a state school or six years apprenticeship with a doctor. Five consecutive years in either a civil or military hospital also were recognized as qualification for this office.

The legal right to practice medicine was based on the acquisition of the degree of officer or doctor and proper registration with civil authorities. The doctorate in medicine required four years of study. The examination included theoretical and practical tests in anatomy, physiology, pathology, nosology, materia medica, chemistry, pharmacology, hygiene, and legal medicine. The terminal thesis had to be written in Latin or French. Medical education developed along two lines: the university, which was fundamental, national, and open to all, and the hospital, which was complimentary and reserved to an elite selected by competition. This system of medical education was to prevail in France until well into the twentieth century. One of the real reasons why Paris was the unquestioned leader of world medicine during the first half of the nineteenth century was the overall reform of its educational system.

Marie-Françoise-Xavier Bichat (1721–1802) is closely associated with the new scientific approach to medicine during the revolutionary period. A surgeon in the revolutionary army, he is regarded as the founder of descriptive anatomy. His *Anatomie Générale* (1801) opened up a new field of pathology with its focus on the study of tissue, arteries, bone, muscle, and glands in the diseased state. During his career, Bichat authored four important studies on systematic anatomy. His "membrane" doctrine, which stated that each tissue had its own vital principle, although now untenable, was a step forward in the study of histology.

The most well known physician of this era was the physician of Napoleon, Jean Nicholas Corvisart (1755–1821). Napoleon once remarked: "I don't believe in medicine but I believe in Corvisart." Yet Napoleon's interest in the promotion of better medical practices must not be underestimated. It is significant that one of his first moves in conquered Egypt was to print on Arabic an account of ophthalmia and manuals on the treatment of bubonic plague and smallpox. He set up quarantine stations throughout the conquered country and erected a three hundred bed hospital for the poor in Cairo. Corvisart authored two books that had a noticeable effect on medicine: *Essai sur les maladies et les lesions du coeur et des vaisseux*, a study of cardiac disease (1806), and the *Reconnaître les maladies internes*, which popularized Auenbrugger's work on percussion.

Corvisart's most famous student was René Theophile Hyacinthe Laennec (1781–1826), perhaps the greatest of the French clinicians. His contribution to the world of medicine was the invention of the stethoscope, which he describes in *De l'auscultation mediate*, published in 1818:

Of all the diseases which are essentially local, those of the thoracic organs are unquestionably the most frequent; while in point of danger they can only be compared with organic affections of the brain. The heart, lungs, and brain constitute, according to the happy expression of Bordeu, the tripod of life; and none of these organs can sustain any considerable or extensive morbid change without the greatest danger. The delicacy of their organization and their incessant motion account for the frequency and severity of their diseases. In no other texture of the animal system is idiopathic and primary inflammation so frequent a source of severe disorder and death as in the lungs; and no other is so liable to become the seat of accidental productions of every kind, more especially of tubercles, the most common of all. The heart, although of a less delicate texture, is equally obnoxious to morbid changes. Of these, it is true, some are only of rare occurrence; but others are extremely common—for instance, thickening of its muscular substance and dilation of its cavities.

Diseases of the chest, in respect of their frequency and severity, hold also the first rank among those affections which, either as complications or effects, are found to accompany other diseases of a general nature. Thus in idiopathic fevers a slight degree of peripneumony, a determination of blood to the lungs, or a catarrh occasioning redness and thickening of the internal membrane of the bronchi and pouring into them an augmented secretion of mucus, are local affections quite as constant in their occurrence as the redness, thickenings or ulcerations of the mucous membrane of the intestines, in which several authors, ancient and modern, have fancied they discovered the cause of these diseases. It may even be asserted that in maladies of every sort, whatever be their seat, death scarcely ever occurs without the chest becoming affected in one way or another; and that, in most cases, life does not seem in peril until the supervention of a congested state of the lungs, serious effusion into the pleura, or a great disorder of the circulation. The brain in general becomes affected only subsequently to these changes; and frequently remains undisturbed even to the last moment of life.

However dangerous diseases of the chest may be, they are, nevertheless, more frequently curable than any other severe internal affection. For this double reason medical men in all ages have been desirous of obtaining a correct diagnosis of them. Hitherto, however, their efforts have been attended by little success, a circumstance which must necessarily result from their having confined their attention to the observation and study of the deranged functions only. From the continued operation of the same cause we must even now confess, with Baglivi, that the diagnosis of the diseases of this cavity is more obscure than that of those of any other internal organ. Diseases of the brain, not in themselves numerous, are distinguished, for the most part, by constant and striking symptoms; the soft and yielding walls of the abdomen allow us to examine, through the medium of touch, the organs of that cavity, and thus to judge, in some measure, of their size, position, and degree of sensibility, and also of the extraneous substances that may be formed in them. On the other hand, the diseases of the thoracic viscera are very numerous and diversified, and yet have almost all the same class of symptoms. Of these, the most common and prominent are cough, dyspnoea, and, in some, expectoration. These, of course, vary in different diseases; but their variations are by no means of that determinate kind which can enable us to consider them as certain indications of known variations in the diseases. The consequence is that the most skillful physician who trusts to the pulse and general symptoms is often deceived in regard to the most common and best known complaints of this cavity. Nay, I will go so far as to assert, and without fear of contradiction from those who have been long accustomed to the examination of dead bodies, that, before the discovery of Auenbrugger, one-half of the acute cases of peripneumony and pleurisy, and almost all the chronic pleurisies, were mistaken by practitioners; and that, in such instances as the superior tact of a physician enabled him to suspect the true nature of the disease, his conviction was rarely sufficiently strong to prompt and justify the application of very powerful remedies. The percussion of the chest, according to the method of the ingenious observer just mentioned, is one of the most valuable discoveries ever made in medicine. By means of it several diseases which had hitherto been cognisable by general and equivocal signs only, are brought within the immediate sphere of our perceptions, and their diagnosis, consequently, rendered both more easy and more certain. It is not to be concealed, however, that this mode of exploration is very incomplete. Confined, in a great measure, to the indication of fulness or emptiness, it is only applicable to a limited number of organic lesions; it does not enable us to discriminate some which are very different in their nature or seat; it scarcely affords any indication except in extreme cases, and cannot, therefore, enable us to detect, or even to suspect, diseases in their very commencement. It is more particularly in diseases of the heart that we regret the insufficiency of this method and wish for something more precise. The general symptoms of disease in this organ greatly resemble those produced by many nervous complaints and by the diseases of other organs. The application of the hand affords some indications as to the extent, strength, and rhythm of the heart's motions; but these in general are by no means distinct, while in cases of considerable fatness or anasarca they become very obscure, or are altogether imperceptible. Within these few years some few physicians have, in those cases, attempted to gain further information by the application of the ear to the cardiac region. In this way the pulsations of the heart, perceived at once by the ear and touch, become, no doubt, more distinct. But even this method comes far short of what might be expected from it. Bayle was the first who, to my knowledge, had recourse to it at the time when we were attending the lectures of Corvisart. This great man himself never used it: he says only that he had several times heard the pulsation of the heart in listening very close to the chest. We shall afterwards find that this phenomenon is different from auscultation, properly so called, and is only observable in some particular cases. But neither Bayle nor any other of our fellow-students, who, with myself, might, in imitation of him, employ this immediate auscultation (of which, by the way, the first notion is derived from Hippocrates), obtained any other result from it than that of perceiving more distinctly the action of the heart, in the cases where this was not very perceptible to the touch. The reason of this limited application will be stated hereafter. But, independently of its deficiencies, there are other objections to its use: it is always inconvenient, both to the physician and patient; in the case of females it is not only indelicate, but often impracticable; and in that class of persons found in hospitals it is disgusting. For these various reasons this measure can but rarely be had recourse to, and cannot, therefore, become practically useful, since it is only by numerous observations and the comparison of numerous facts of the same kind that we can ever, in medicine, separate the truth from the errors which are constantly derived from the inexperience of the observer, from the varying fitness of his perceptive powers, the illusions of his senses, and the inherent difficulties of the method of exploration which he employs. Observations made after long intervals can never overcome difficulties of this kind. Nevertheless, I had been in the habit of using this method for a long time, in obscure cases, and where it was practicable; and it was the employment of it which led me to the discovery of one much better.

In 1816 I was consulted by a young woman labouring under general symptoms of diseased heart, and in whose case percussion and the application of the hand were of little avail on account of the great degree of fatness. The other method just mentioned being rendered inadmissible by the age and sex of the patient, I happened to recollect a simple well-known fact in acoustics, and fancied it might be turned to some use on the present occasion. The fact I allude to is the great distinctness with which we hear the scratch of a pin at one end of a piece of wood on applying our ear to the other. Immediately, on this suggestion, I rolled a quire of paper into a kind of cylinder and applied one end of it to the region of the heart and the other to my ear, and was not a little surprised and pleased to find that I could thereby perceive the action of the heart in a manner much more clear and distinct than I had ever been able to do by the immediate application of the ear.

Not all was brilliance at the famous Paris school, however. François Broussais (1772–1838), who served for three years as a surgeon in Napoleon's armies, created a sanguine vogue throughout France by curing diseases through massive applications of leeches. It is estimated that in the year 1833 more than 41 million leeches were imported into France because of Broussais' cure-all methods.

German-born Franz Joseph Gall (1758–1828) also led many astray with his phrenological doctrines. He taught that the cranium was the only faithful cast of the external surface of the brain. His efforts to localize mental functions and diseases by "cranioscopy," although erroneous, did eventually lead to a more fruitful investigation of the anatomy of the brain.

Two figures tower above all others in mid-nineteeth-century France: Claude Bernard (1813–78) and Louis Pasteur (1822–95). Neither were practicing physicians; yet both profoundly changed medical science. Bernard, like so many other prominent men of medicine in postrevolutionary France, was of humble rural origins. After studying pharmacy in Lyons, he turned to playwriting and enjoyed minor success in Paris. Advised that medicine would provide a better livelihood than the Muses, he became an apprentice to the famed Françoise Magendie (1783–1855) at the College de France. Magendie was the most respected physiologist in Paris at this time and had carried out extensive experiments in the mechanics of digestion and the role of the spinal nerves. These studies were to be continued and perfected by his much more systematic student. Bernard received a doctorate in medicine in 1843. His thesis proved that when cane sugar is injected into the vein it appears in the urine if it is not previously treated with gastric juice. He later elaborated this discovery by demonstrating that pancreatic juices aided digestion by acting on fats, proteins, and starches. Later contributions were his discovery of the glycogenetic function of the liver and the demonstration of the vasomotor mechanism. Because the vasomotor nerves regulate the dilation and contraction of the walls of the blood vessels, this discovery led to great advances in psychology as well as physiology. Among Bernard's lesser but none the less important discoveries was the poisonous effect of carbon monoxide and the role of the red blood cells in respiration. Other experiments were to lead to modern notions on metabolism and the role of the ductless glands.

Toward the end of his career, Bernard became embroiled in an academic dispute about spontaneous generation. His antagonist in this debate was the most striking figure in nineteenth-century medicine—Louis Pasteur.

Pasteur was, like Bernard, of humble background; he was the son of a tanner in Dole. Also like Bernard, he received a well-rounded education. After taking a bachelor of science degree in 1842 from the College of Bescençon, he studied at the Ecole Normale in Paris. He first interested himself in one of the chemical dilemmas of the day—the fact that certain substances, although composed of the same ingredients, exhibited different physical and chemical qualities. In 1841, German chemist Eilhard Mitscherlich had announced that certain salts, the tartrates and paratartrates of soda and ammonia, although possessing the same crystalline form, nevertheless caused different reactions when dissolved in water. The tartaric acid rotated the plane of polarized light, while the paratartric acid remained inactive. This principle of isomorphism was further explained by Pasteur, who found that the paratartrates were actually composed of crystals that were dissymmetrical, that is, whose images reflected in a mirror cannot be superposed on the crystals themselves. Pasteur's discovery was immediately taken up by the French Academy of Science, and its repercussions were sensational. Not only did Pasteur lay the foundation for sterochemistry but he also provided evidence that products of vegetable and animal life are dissymmetrical.

In 1854, after having taught in Dijon and Strasbourg, he was appointed dean of the science faculty at Lille. There he turned from the study of crystals to fermentation, considered at that time to be a chemical process. By studying alcoholic and lactic fermentation, he concluded that ferments are living cells, that they originate only from cells of the same species, and that fermentation is impossible in their absence. The demonstration proved a death blow to the idea of spontaneous generation, for Pasteur showed that microscopic organisms were introduced by the air. Pasteur's studies in fermentation led him naturally to the study of disease. During the early 1860s, the lucrative silk industry in France was almost completely destroyed by a mysterious disease that infected the silkworms. Pasteur, after extensive study, showed that the disease was caused, not by one identified disease entity, pebrine, but by another as well, flacherie, which affected the intestines of the worms.

Following his success at saving the silk industry, Pasteur turned his attentions to two other facets of French industry—beer and wine. Here he demonstrated that by heating them to a temperature of between 50° and 60° Centigrade the spoilage could be drastically reduced. There was an element of chauvinism in Pasteur's desire that France produce a superior beer. As an extremely patriotic Frenchman, he saw the defeat of France in the Franco-Prussian War as a reversal of civilization. So much so that he returned to the University of Bonn a medical degree that it had awarded him in 1868. Between 1871 and 1885, Pasteur discovered preventive inoculation, produced vaccines against chicken cholera and anthrax, and developed a cure for hydrophobia. In the following passage, he discusses the germ theory and its applications to medicine and surgery:

The Sciences gain by mutual support. When, as the result of my first communications on the fermentations in 1857-1858, it appeared that the ferments, properly so-called, are living beings, that the germs of microscopic organisms abound in the surface of all objects, in the air and in water; that the theory of spontaneous generation is chimerical; that wines, beer, vinegar, the blood, urine and all the fluids of the body undergo none of their usual changes in pure air, both Medicine and Surgery received fresh stimulation. A French physician, Dr. Davaine, was fortunate in making the first application of these principles to Medicine, in 1863.

Our researches of last year, left the etiology of the putrid disease, or septicemis, in a much less advanced condition than that of anthrax. We had demonstrated the probability that septicemia depends upon the presence and growth of a microscopic body, but the absolute proof of this important conclusion was not reached. To demonstrate experimentally that a microscopic organism actually is the cause of a disease and the agent of contagion, I know no other way, in the present state of Science, than to subject the microbe (the new and happy term introduced by M. Sedillot) to the method of cultivation out of the body. It may be noted that in twelve successive cultures, each one of only ten cubic centimeters volume, the original drop will be diluted as if placed in a volume of fluid equal to the total volume of the earth. It is just this form of test to which M. Joubert and I subjected the anthrax bacteridium. Having cultivated it a great number of times, in a sterile fluid, each culture being started with a minute drop from the preceding, we then demonstrated that the product of the last culture was capable of further development and of acting in the animal tissues by producing anthrax with all its symptoms. Such is—as we believe—the indisputable proof that *anthrax is a bacterial disease.*

Our researches concerning the septic vibrio had not so far been convincing, and it was to fill up this gap that we resumed our experiments. To this end, we attempted the cultivation of the septic vibrio from an animal dead of septicemia. It is worth noting that all of our first experiments failed, despite the variety of culture media we employed—urine, beer yeast water, meat water, etc. Our culture media were not sterile, but we found—most commonly a microscopic organism showing no relationship to the septic vibrio, and presenting the form, common enough elsewhere, of chains of extremely minute spherical granules possessed of no virulence whatever. This was an impurity, introduced, unknown to us, at the same time as the septic vibrio; and the germ undoubtedly passed from the intestines—always inflamed and distended in septicemic animals—into the abdominal fluids from which we took our original cultures of the septic vibrio. If this explanation of the contamination of our cultures was correct, we ought to find a pure culture of the septic vibrio in the heart's blood of an animal recently dead of septicemia. This was what happened, but a new difficulty presented itself; all our cultures remained sterile. Furthermore this sterility was accompanied by loss in the culture media of [the original] virulence.

It occurred to us that the septic vibrio might be an obligatory anaërobe and that the sterility of our inoculated culture fluids might be due to the destruction of the septic vibrio by the atmospheric oxygen dissolved in the fluids. The Academy may remember that I have previously demonstrated facts of this nature in regard to the vibrio of butyric fermentation, which not only lives without air but is killed by the air.

It was necessary therefore to attempt to cultivate the septic vibrio either in a vacuum or in the presence of inert gases—such as carbonic acid.

Results justified our attempt; the septic vibrio grew easily in a complete vacuum, and no less easily in the presence of pure carbonic acid.

These results have a necessary corollary. If a fluid containing septic vibrios be exposed to pure air, the vibrios should be killed and all virulence should disappear. This is actually the case. If some drops of septic serum be spread horizontally in a tube and in a very thin layer, the fluid will become absolutely harmless in less than half a day, even if at first it was so virulent as to produce death upon the inoculation of the smallest portion of a drop.

Furthermore all the vibrios, which crowded the liquid as motile threads, are destroyed, and disappear. After the action of the air, only fine amorphous granules can be found, unfit for culture as well as for the transmission of any disease whatever. It might be said that the air burned the vibrios.

If it is a terrifying thought that life is at the mercy of the multiplication of these minute bodies, it is a consoling hope that Science will not always remain powerless before such enemies, since for example at the very beginning of the study we find that simple exposure to air is sufficient at times to destroy them.

But if oxygen destroys the vibrios, how can septicemia exist, since atmospheric air is present everywhere? How can such facts be brought in accord with the germ theory? How can blood, exposed to air, become septic through the dust the air contains?

All things are hidden, obscure and debatable if the cause of the phenomena be unknown, but everything is clear if this cause be known. What we have just said is true only of a septic fluid containing adult vibrios, in active development by fission: conditions are different when the vibrios are transformed into their germs, that is into the glistening corpuscles first described and figured in my studies on silk-worm disease, in dealing with worms dead of the disease called "flacherie." Only the adult vibrios disappear, burn up, and lose their virulence in contact with air: the germ corpuscles, under these conditions, remain always ready for new cultures, and for new inoculations.

All this however does not do away with the difficulty of understanding how septic germs can exist on the surface of objects, floating in the air and in water.

Where can these corpuscles originate? Nothing is easier than the production of these germs, in spite of the presence of air in contact with septic fluids.

If abdominal serous exudate containing septic vibrios actively growing by fission be exposed to the air, as we suggested above, but with the precaution of giving a substantial thickness to the layer, even if only one centimeter be used, this curious phenomenon will appear in a few hours. The oxygen is absorbed in the upper layers of the fluid—as is indicated by the change of color. Here the vibrios are dead and disappear. In the deeper layers, on the other hand, towards the bottom of this centimeter of septic fluid we suppose to be under observation, the vibrios continue to multiply by fission—protected from the action of oxygen by those that have perished above them: little by little they pass over to the condition of germ corpuscles with the gradual disappearance of the thread forms. So that instead of moving threads of varying length, sometimes greater than the field of the microscope, there is to be seen only a number of glittering points, lying free or surrounded by a scarcely perceptible amorphous mass. Thus is formed, containing the latent germ life, no longer in danger from the destructive action of oxygen, thus, I repeat, is formed the septic dust, and we are able to understand what has before seemed so obscure; we can see how putrescible fluids can be inoculated by the dust of the air, and how it is that putrid diseases are permanent in the world. (*Comptes Rendus de l'Académie des Sciences,* IXXXVI)

By the middle of the nineteenth century, leadership in medical science had shifted from France to Germany. Once again, it was superiority in university education that was a decisive factor in this move. The reforms in German education inaugurated in 1809 by Wilhelm von Humboldt (1767–1835) produced a dramatic change that soon brought the German universities to the forefront of higher education in Europe. Humboldt's basic creed, that science be considered an organic totality and that it be approached by critical methods, was combined with a new idea of academic freedom and personal self-education. Research and teaching were combined because only the productive scholar can truly further the cause of knowledge. Inspired by the high ideal that the instructor would not only inform the student through his creative scholarship but inspire him to personal self-education, the University of Berlin was opened in 1810. Soon thereafter, the University of Bonn was established in the Rhineland, and within the next decade, the new academic style was adopted in other universities throughout the German states. Thus, unlike Austria and France, where the centers of medical study remained localized in Vienna and Paris, the new German experiment was spread throughout the various German states. By the end of the century, German scholarship had become the model for scientific research throughout the world.

Two names stand out among the physician-scientists who were to elevate Germany to a pinnacle of excellence: Johann Schonlein and Johannes Muller. Schonlein (1793–1864), who received his medical degree from the University of Wurzburg in 1816 and held chairs of medicine there as well as at Zurich and Berlin, was the first to combine clinical demonstration and scientific experimentation. It is significant that his lectures were delivered in German rather than the traditional Latin. Schonlein's reputation was based on his teaching ability rather than on his writings. He was the first to describe Peliosis rheumatica, and he discovered the parasitic cause of fauvus. In Berlin, he was the personal physician to the king of Prussia and counselor to the Ministry of Education.

Johannes Muller (1801–58) graduated from the University of Bonn in 1822 and held a chair as professor of anatomy and physiology there until he was called to Berlin in 1833. He collaborated with Schonlein in making Berlin one of the great centers of medical study. The student enrollment in medicine rose from 397 in 1819 to 1,568 in 1909, the faculty from 28 to 202. The two men developed a new concept of research that combined laboratory and clinical work. The end result was that education in the natural sciences became an absolute necessity for the medical student. The combining of the sciences and the clinic with the resulting specialization forms the basis of modern medicine.

Muller's contribution to this new approach cannot be overestimated, for he was equally familiar with biology, embryology, comparative anatomy, physiology, chemistry, psychology, and pathology. His many discoveries include the true nature of reflex actions, the isolation of chondrin and glutin, Muller's ducts, the metamorphosis of ecinodermata, the identity of the pathological and embryonic development of tumors, and the basic law of specific nerve energy. The journal that he founded in 1834, *Archiv für Anatomie und Psychologie,* is regarded as one of the most important publications in nineteenth-century medicine. It would not be incorrect to speak of Muller as a nineteenth-century Boerhaave, for his students formed the elite of Germany's medical scientists: Theodore Schwann (1810–82), co-founder of the cell theory; Rudolf Virchow (1821–1902), father of modern pathology; and Hermann von Helmholtz (1821–94), founder of the law of conservation of energy.

Schwann was born in the Ruhr city of Neuss and studied under Muller at Bonn and Berlin, where he graduated in 1834. His doctoral thesis demonstrated the necessity of oxygen for the egg embryo. He was later to discover the sheath of the axis cylinder of the nerves, the striped muscle in the upper esophagus, and the role of the enzyme pepsin in digestion. However, his greatest claim to fame was his discovery, in collaboration with Matthias Schleiden (1804–81), of the cell theory, and he is thus regarded as the founder of histology. As was the case in so many other scientific breakthroughs, there were a number of concurrent studies of the cells in animals and plants. However, the publication in 1839 of Schwann's *Microscopical Researches into the Accordance in Structure and Growth of Plants and Animals,* which demonstrated that both plants and animals are composed of cells and that the cells of each tissue have their own characteristics, gave most of the credit to the German physician. Schwann left the University of Berlin in 1839 and spent the remainder of his career in Belgium, lecturing at the universities of Louvain and Liège.

The theory discovered by Schwann and Schleiden was further developed and applied to pathology by Rudolf Virchow. Born in Pomerania, Virchow graduated with a medical degree from the University of Berlin in 1843. His liberal political views and his deep concern over the wretched working conditions brought to Germany by the Industrial Revolution alienated him from Prussian officialdom, and he left Berlin for Wurzburg, where he remained for seven years, returning to Berlin in 1856. During these years, he discovered leukemia and introduced the terms "embolism" and "thrombosis." Two years later,

he published his epoch-making *Cellular Pathology,* which was to revo-
lutionize medical thinking on disease. The body was a cell society in
which every cell was a citizen. Disease was a conflict of the citizens
caused from outside. His famous dictum was *omnis cellula e cellula*—
every cell from a cell. In other words, a new growth of cells presupposes already existing cells. Here, in his own words, is how Virchow
describes his all-important discovery:

What Schwann, however, has done for histology, has as yet been in a very
slight degree built up and developed for pathology and it may be said that
nothing has penetrated less deeply into the minds of all than the cell-theory
in its intimate connection with pathology.

If we consider the extraordinary influence which Bichat in his time exercised upon the state of medical opinion, it is indeed astonishing that such a
relatively long period should have elapsed since Schwann made his great
discoveries, without the real importance of the new facts having been duly
appreciated. This has certainly been essentially due to the great incomplete-
ness of our knowledge with regard to the intimate structure of our tissues
which has continued to exist until quite recently, and, as we are sorry to be
obliged to confess, still even now prevails with regard to many points of
histology to such a degree, that we scarcely know in favour of what to decide.

Especial difficulty has been found in answering the question, from what
parts of the body action really proceeds—what parts are active, what passive;
and yet it is already quite possible to come to a definitive conclusion upon
this point, even in the case of parts the structure of which is still disputed.
The chief point in this application of histology to pathology is to obtain a
recognition of the fact, that the cell is really the ultimate morphological
element in which there is any manifestation of life, and that we must not
transfer the seat of real action to any point beyond the cell. Before you, I shall
offer no particular reason to justify myself, if in this respect I make a quite
special reservation in favour of life. But I think that we must look upon this
as certain, that, however much of the more delicate interchange of matter,
which takes place within a cell, may not concern the material structure as a
whole, yet the real action does proceed from the structure as such, and that
the living element only maintains its activity as long as it really presents itself
to us as an independent whole.

In this question it is of primary importance (and you will excuse my
dwelling a little upon this point, as it is one which is still a matter of dispute)
that we should determine what is really to be understood by the term cell.
Quite at the beginning of the latest phase of histological development, great
difficulties sprang up in crowds with regard to this matter. Schwann, as you

no doubt recollect, following immediately in the footsteps of Schleiden, interpreted his observations according to botanical standards, so that all the doctrines of vegetable physiology were invoked, in a greater or less degree, to decide questions relating to the physiology of animal bodies. Vegetable cells, however, in the light in which they were at that time universally, and as they are even now also frequently regarded, are structures, whose identity with what we call animal cells cannot be admitted without reserve.

It is only when we adhere to this view of the matter, when we separate from the cell all that has been added to it by an after-development, that we obtain a simple, homogeneous, extremely monotonous structure, recurring with extraordinary constancy in living organisms. But just this very constancy forms the best criterion of our having before us in this structure one of those really elementary bodies, to be built up of which is eminently characteristic of every living thing—without the pre-existence of which no living forms arise, and to which continuance and the maintenance of life is intimately attached. Only since our idea of a cell has assumed this severe form—and I am somewhat proud of having always, in spite of the reproach of pedantry, firmly adhered to it—only since that time can it be said that a simple form has been obtained which we can everywhere again expect to find, and which, though different in size and external shape, is yet always identical in its essential constituents.

Hermann von Helmholtz received his medical degree at the University of Berlin in 1842. Five years later, he achieved international fame with his discovery of the law of conservation of energy. Combining the interests of the physicist and the physician, he revived the Thomas Young (1773–1820) theory of color vision, which is due to retinal structures corresponding to red, green, and violet. He also measured the velocity of nervous impulses and demonstrated that muscles are the chief source of animal heat. By inventing the ophthalmoscope and the phakoscope, he revolutionized ophthalmology.

Although Virchow dominated German medicine during the latter half of the century, distinguishing himself as an historian and an anthropologist, it was Robert Koch (1843–1910) who caught the attention of the entire world because of his work in bacteriology. Following his graduation from Göttingen in 1866, he served for a time as an army surgeon during the Franco-Prussian War. He spent the next decade in relative seclusion in rural Wollstein, working on the process of developing various bacilli. In 1876, he demonstrated that pure cultures of anthrax could cause the disease when injected into animals by means of sporulation. His experiments had definitely proven that pure cultures, grown through several generations, can produce disease when injected into living beings. Shortly thereafter, he disclosed a practical method for fixing and staining bacterial films. In 1881, the year after his appointment to the Imperial Health Office in Berlin, he demonstrated his new method for obtaining pure cultures of bacteria by using a meat infusion mixed with warm gelatin. His discovery of the tubercle bacillus in 1882 and the cholera vibrio a year later marked the beginning of a new era in medical history. By the end of the century, the bacteria that caused diphtheria, tetanus, botulism, and plague had been discovered. In addition, progress was made in defining organisms so small that they could not be detected by ordinary microscopes. They were termed "viruses." Koch continued his work until his death in 1910. In 1905, he received the Nobel prize; yet his final years were marred by the scandal of his marriage to eighteen-year-old Hedwig Freiberg, a girl he had met in a Berlin *atelier.* In the following selection, Koch writes of the etiology of tuberculosis:

The question whether tuberculosis is due to a virus communicable from man to man can be approached in various ways, as has actually been the case. Clinical observation, anatomical, and latterly experimental, investigation have each in turn been called in to furnish information as to the true nature of this disease.

The least satisfactory results have been furnished by observations at the bedside. Cases occur now and then to every physician in even moderately extensive practice, in which he cannot do otherwise than assume that an infection of one person by another suffering from tuberculosis has taken place. Against these, however, may be set numerous instances where every possibility of infection seems to be excluded. The attempt has again and again been made to prove on the evidence of such collected clinical observations that phthisis is contagious, but the theory thus supported has met with no acceptance in the scientific world, and the attempt must be regarded as a failure. Many practical men have no doubt kept in mind the possibility of infection, but with the medical profession generally, phthisis is regarded as the result of constitutional peculiarities rather than of direct contagion.

Pathological anatomy bore an unimportant testimony to the infectious nature of tuberculosis when Buhl drew attention to the connection between military tuberculosis and primary cheesy foci, and propounded the theory that general tuberculosis must be regarded as a disease due to the absorption of a virus originally present in the primary cheesy nodule, and thus depending to a certain extent on self-infection. As to the way in which the virus of tubercle spreads through the body, much information was afforded by Ponfick's discoveries with regard to tuberculosis of the thoracic duct, and Weigert's detection of tubercle in the walls of veins in military tuberculosis. These facts, however, bear only upon the diffusion of the tubercular virus within the body; we cannot conclude from them that the virus is communicable from one individual to another, or, in other words, that the disease is truly infectious.

With the latter question experimental pathology has dealt in the most exact way. The course of experimental research into the infective nature of tuberculosis has lately been fully considered on several occasions (S. Johne, *Die Geschichte der Tuberkulose,* Leipzig, 1883), so that I shall limit myself to a few remarks on the points of most importance.

Isolated, imperfect attempts at the artificial production of tuberculosis made at the end of the last century gave only negative results. The credit of the first successful experiments belongs to Klencke, who in the year 1843 succeeded in inducing an extensive tuberculosis of the lungs and liver in rabbits, by inoculation with portions of military and infiltrating tubercles from Man; and he did this by the introduction of these masses into the veins of the neck. He did not continue his researches, and they were consequently soon forgotten. In the meantime Villemin undertook an experimental investigation into the nature of tuberculosis, working in a methodical and thorough manner. He inoculated not only with tubercular material from human beings, but also from cases of bovine tuberculosis, and proved experimentally the identity of the latter disease with human tuberculosis. Villemin's researches, from the number of his experiments, the careful manner in which they were carried out and the employment of suitable control experiments, appeared to have decided the question in favour of the infective theory. The numerous workers, however, who repeated Villemin's experiments after the same or a modified method, arrived at very contradictory results. The partisans of the infective theory, amongst whom Klebs must be specially noticed, sought to improve the details of the experimental method and to free it from the imperfections surrounding it; its opponents strove, on the contrary, to prove that tubercular material contained no specific virus, and that true tuberculosis could be induced by inoculation with non-tubercular material. To the decision of this question Cohnheim and Salomonsen contributed largely by selecting for inoculation, in a moment of inspiration, the anterior chamber of a rabbit's eye. By this means it is possible to separate the cases in which successful inoculation with tubercular material has been accomplished from those in which some other infective material has been introduced with the tubercular virus. Subcutaneous inoculation with such material often causes a more or less widely diffused cheesy infiltration, not unlike that of tubercle. But in the eye these substances give rise only to a general inflammation of short duration, which cannot in any case be mistaken for the slow and characteristic development of tuberculosis resulting from inoculation. The course of a successful tubercular inoculation can be watched throughout by the experimenter. After a fairly long incubation period, single grey nodules, barely visible to the naked eye, appear in the iris, starting from the piece of material introduced. The number of nodules gradually increases, they enlarge, become yellowish in the centre, caseate, and show macroscopically as well as microscopically all the typical characters of the true tubercular nodule. The tubercular infection, however, does not remain limited to the eye, but invades later the whole organism, spreading to the neighbouring lymphatic glands, the lungs, spleen, liver and kidneys. Cohnheim and Salomonsen, as also the observers who repeated their experiments, unanimously state that in no case did tuberculosis of the iris follow an inoculation with non-tubercular material. A further point is that spontaneous tuberculosis of the iris has never been observed in rabbits. This method of infection, is, therefore, preferable to all others, in so far as it completely excludes both a vitiation of the experiment by unnoticed errors of manipulation, such as may easily occur in cases of subcutaneous inoculation or introduction of materials into the peritoneal cavity, and also the possibility of mistaking spontaneous tuberculosis for an artificially induced form of the disease. In contradistinction to the earlier experiments on the infective nature of tubercle, the researches of Cohnheim and Salomonsen must, therefore, be regarded as quite free from objection, and they established the fact that tubercular materials, apparently differing widely from each other, are characterized by one and the same specific contagium. But it was impossible at the time to decide upon the nature of this contagium—whether it consisted of independent organisms, endowed with constant properties, which invaded the body as parasites and rendered it tubercular, or whether it was composed of particles of an organized or even unorganized nature, arising only under certain abnormal conditions within the body and indeed from its own elements.

Judging from the results which had been recently attained concerning the etiology of many infective diseases, it seemed not unlikely that the cause of tuberculosis might also be found in some micro-organism. To arrive at some conclusion on this point, it was obviously necessary to utilize all those methods which had proved of value in the investigation of other infective diseases, and to follow that order of research which had on former occasions proved itself best adapted to the end in view. Consequently, the following plan in inquiry was decided upon. First, to determine whether formed elements, which could neither belong to the constituents of the body, nor have sprung from them, were present in the diseased parts. Were the presence of such foreign elements demonstrated, it would next be necessary to ascertain whether they were organized, and whether they exhibited any signs of possessing independent life, the chief of these being spontaneous movement, so often confounded with molecular motion, the power of growth, increase, and reproduction. Further, the relations of these forms to their surroundings, the behaviour of the neighbouring tissue-elements, the distribution of these forms through the body, their presence in different stages of the morbid process, and similar points, would have to be worked out; these all having a bearing of more or less importance on the causal relation of these forms to the disease under consideration. It seemed possible that the facts thus brought to light might furnish such decisive proof, that only the most extreme sceptic would still maintain that the micro-organisms discovered were concomitants, and not the cause, of the disease. Often, however, there may be grounds for this objection; complete proof of the causal relationship demands, not merely a demonstration of the coincidence of the parasites with the disease, but, beyond this, it must be shown that the parasites directly produce the disease. To obtain this proof, it is necessary to isolate the parasites completely from the diseased organism, and from all the products of the disease to which any pathogenic influence could be ascribed; then to excite anew the disease with all its special characteristics by the introduction of the parasites alone into a healthy organism.

While the British Isles lagged behind the continent in medical achievement, there were notable exceptions. Unlike France and Germany, where the universities were the centers for the new training that combined lecture, laboratory, and clinic, England produced most of its practicing physicians through training at private hospital schools. The system was in essence an extension of the old apprenticeship method. Until the Apothecaries Act of 1815, the actual licensing of medical practitioners was not required by law. Medical education at Oxford and Cambridge had fallen to new lows during the early nineteenth century. The most famous of the hospital doctors were associated with Guy's Hospital in London. Richard Bright (1789–1858) was educated at Edinburgh and in 1820 began his medical career at Guy's, where he was to remain for the next forty years. He first achieved fame through the publication of *Reports on Medical Cases* (1827). Here he described and illustrated the relation between diseased kidneys, dropsy, and albuminous urine and defined the disease still known by his name.

Thomas Addison (1793–1860), who served on the staff of Guy's for thirty-six years, is known for his description of *melasma suprarenale,* the bronzed skin associated with the suprarenal glands, or, as it is now known, Addison's disease. He was also the first to describe pernicious anemia and xanthoma diabeticorum. Thomas Hodgkin (1798–1866), who graduated from Edinburgh in 1823, is known for his description of the simultaneous enlargement of the spleen and lymphatic glands, known as Hodgkin's disease.

Mention must also be made of the Irish school of medicine, which achieved considerable fame during the nineteenth century. Robert Graves (1796–1853) introduced continental practices into the Meath Hospital in Dublin and was especially known for his treatment of fevers. William Stokes (1804–78) specialized in diseases of the chest and of the heart and aorta. In 1825, he published *The Use of the Stethoscope,* the first description of the new instrument published in England. Dominic Corrigan (1820–80) is recalled because of his description of "Corrigan's pulse," associated with insufficiency of the aortic valve.

Perhaps the most significant British contribution to medical progress during the nineteenth century was the discovery of antiseptics by Quaker physician Joseph Lister (1827–1912). Educated at the newly founded University of London, he spent most of his career as professor of surgery, first at the University of Glasgow and later at Edinburgh. Inspired by Pasteur's discoveries about the true nature of putrefaction, he thought of using carbolic acid as an antiseptic. Beginning with the application of this solution for open fractures, he soon applied it to all types of surgery. By the end of the century, the horrors of hospital gangrene had been greatly reduced, and survival after major surgery became a reality. Here is Lister's own description of the "antiseptic principle":

In the course of an extended investigation into the nature of inflammation, and the healthy and morbid conditions of the blood in relation to it, I arrived several years ago at the conclusion that the essential cause of suppuration in wounds is decomposition brought about by the influence of the atmosphere upon blood or serum retained within them, and, in the case of contused wounds, upon portions of tissue destroyed by the violence of the injury.

To prevent the occurrence of suppuration with all its attendant risks was an object manifestly desirable, but till lately apparently unattainable, since it seemed hopeless to attempt to exclude the oxygen which was universally regarded as the agent by which putrefaction was effected. But when it had been shown by the researchers of Pasteur that the septic properties of the atmosphere depended not on the oxygen, or any gaseous constituent, but on minute organisms suspended in it, which owed their energy to their vitality, it occurred to me that decomposition in the injured part might be avoided without excluding the air, by applying as a dressing some material capable of destroying the life of the floating particles. Upon this principle I have based a practice of which I will now attempt to give a short account.

The material which I have employed is carbolic or phenic acid, a volatile organic compound, which appears to exercise a peculiarly destructive influence upon low forms of life, and hence is the most powerful antiseptic with which we are at present acquainted.

The first class of cases to which I applied it was that of compound fractures, in which the effects of decomposition in the injured part were especially striking and pernicious. The results have been such as to establish conclusively the great principle that all local inflammatory mischief and general febrile disturbances which follow severe injuries are due to the irritating and poisonous influence of decomposing blood or sloughs. For these evils are entirely avoided by the antiseptic treatment, so that limbs which would otherwise be unhesitatingly condemned to amputation may be retained, with confidence of the best results.

In conducting the treatment, the first object must be the destruction of any septic germs which may have been introduced into the wounds, either at the moment of the accident or during the time which has since elapsed. This is done by introducing the acid of full strength into all accessible recesses of the wound by means of a piece of rag held in dressing forceps and dipped into the liquid. This I did not venture to do in the earlier cases; but experience has shown that the compound which carbolic acid forms with the blood, and also any portions of tissue killed by its caustic action, including even parts of the bone, are disposed of by absorption and organisation, provided they are afterwards kept from decomposing. We are thus enabled to employ the antiseptic treatment efficiently at a period after the occurrence of the injury at which it would otherwise probably fail. Thus I have now under my care, in Glasgow Infirmary, a boy who was admitted with compound fracture of the leg as late as eight and one-half hours after the accident, in whom, nevertheless, all local and constitutional disturbance was avoided by means of carbolic acid, and the bones were soundly united five weeks after his admission.

The next object to be kept in view is to guard effectually against the spreading of decomposition into the wound along the stream of blood and serum which oozes out during the first few days after the accident, when the acid originally applied has been washed out or dissipated by absorption and evaporation. This part of the treatment has been greatly improved during the past few weeks. The method which I have hitherto published (see *Lancet* for Mar. 16th, 23rd, 30th, and April 27th of the present year) consisted in the application of a piece of lint dipped in the acid, overlapping the sound skin to some extent and covered with a tin cap, which was daily raised in order to touch the surface of the lint with the antiseptic. This method certainly succeeded well with wounds of moderate size; and indeed I may say that in all the many cases of this kind which have been so treated by myself or my house-surgeons, not a single failure has occurred. When, however, the wound is very large, the flow of blood and serum is so profuse, especially during the first twenty-four hours, that the antiseptic application cannot prevent the spread of decomposition into the interior unless it overlaps the sound skin for a very considerable distance, and this was inadmissible by the method described above, on account of the extensive sloughing of the surface of the cutis which it would involve. This difficulty has, however, been overcome by employing a paste composed of common whiting (carbonate of lime), mixed with a solution of one part of carbolic acid in four parts of boiled linseed oil so as to form a firm putty. This application contains the acid in too dilute a form to excoriate the skin, which it may be made to cover to any extent that may be thought desirable, while its substance serves as a reservoir of the antiseptic material. So long as any discharge continues, the paste should be changed daily, and, in order to prevent the chance of mischief occurring during the process, a piece of rag dipped in the solution of carbolic acid in oil is put on next the skin, and maintained there permanently, care being taken to avoid raising it along with the putty. This rag is always kept in an antiseptic condition from contact with the paste above it, and destroys any germs which may fall upon it during the short time that should alone be allowed to pass in the changing of the dressing. The putty should be in a layer about a quarter of an inch thick, and may be advantageously applied rolled out between two pieces of thin calico, which maintain it in the form of a continuous sheet, which may be wrapped in a moment round the whole circumference of a limb if this be thought desirable, while the putty is prevented by the calico from sticking to the rag which is next the skin. When all discharge has ceased, the use of the paste is discontinued, but the original rag is left adhering to the skin till healing by scabbing is supposed to be complete. I have at present in the hospital a man with severe compound fracture of both bones of the left leg, caused by direct violence, who after the cessation of the sanious discharge under the use of the paste, without a drop of pus appearing, has been treated for the last two weeks exactly as if the fracture was a simple one. During this time the rag, adhering by means of a crust of inspissated blood collected beneath it, has continued perfectly dry, and it will be left untouched till the usual period for removing the splints in a simple fracture, when we may fairly expect to find a sound cicatrix beneath it.

We cannot, however, always calculate on so perfect a result as this. More or less pus may appear after the lapse of the first week, and the larger the wound, the more likely this is to happen. And here I would desire earnestly to enforce the necessity of persevering with the antiseptic application in spite of the appearance of suppuration, so long as other symptoms are favorable. The surgeon is extremely apt to suppose that any suppuration is an indication that the antiseptic treatment has failed, and that poulticing or water dressing should be resorted to. But such a course would in many cases sacrifice a limb or a life. I cannot, however, expect my professional brethren to follow my advice blindly in such a matter, and therefore I feel it necessary to place before them, as shortly as I can, some pathological principles intimately connected, not only with the point we are immediately considering, but with the whole subject of this paper.

If a perfectly healthy granulating sore be well washed and covered with a plate of clean metal, such as block tin, fitting its surface pretty accurately, and overlapping the surrounding skin an inch or so in every direction and retained in position by adhesive plaster and a bandage, it will be found, on removing it after twenty-four or forty-eight hours, that little or nothing that can be called pus is present, merely a little transparent fluid, while at the same time there is an entire absence of the unpleasant odour invariably perceived when water dressing is changed. Here the clean metallic surface presents no recesses like those of porous lint for the septic germs to develop in, the fluid exuding from the surface of the granulations has flowed away undecomposed, and the result is the absence of suppuration. This simple experiment illustrates the important fact that granulations have no inherent tendency to form pus, but do so only when subjected to preternatural stimulus. Further, it shows that the mere contact of a foreign body does not of itself stimulate granulations to suppurate: whereas the presence of decomposing organic matter does. These truths are even more strikingly exemplified by the fact that I have elsewhere recorded (*Lancet,* March 23rd, 1867), that a piece of dead bone free from decomposition may not only fail to induce the granulations around it to suppurate, but may actually be absorbed by them; whereas a bit of dead bone soaked with putrid pus infallibly induces suppuration in its vicinity.

While the introduction of effective antiseptics did much to reduce the risks involved in surgery, the discovery of a practical method of anesthesia greatly reduced popular abhorrence of the knife. Although the use of ether had been recommended late in the nineteenth century as an anesthetic by Sir Humphrey Davy (1778–1829), it was not until 1842 that a successful operation was carried out using ether for this purpose. In that year, Crawford W. Long (1815–78) of Danville, Georgia, removed a tumor from the neck of a patient anesthetized with ether. The same year also witnessed the extraction of a tooth by Elijah Pope in Rochester, New York. The first public demonstration of surgical anesthesia took place four years later in Boston, under the direction of William Norton (1819–68). These events were milestones in the gradual evolution of American medicine.

Another of the major advances of the nineteenth century that led to significant changes in the care of the sick was the development of nursing as a respectable lay vocation. This was almost entirely due to the dedicated work of one woman: Florence Nightingale.

In the Middle Ages, monasteries were opened to the sick, and convents accepted the responsibility for their care. The abbess Hildegarde of Rupertsburg organized a nursing school in the latter part of the twelfth century, and the great orders of religieuses of today, dedicated to nursing and other charitable works, have their roots in fourteenth-century foundations.

In the first half of the nineteenth century, apart from the religious orders, the servant-nurses in European hospitals were usually drunken and dissolute women, and many of them were prostitutes. In 1840, the beginnings of reform appeared in London with the organization of Mrs. Fry's Protestant Nursing Sisters to care for the destitute, but significant change did not occur until the time of Florence Nightingale.

Florence Nightingale (1820–1910) was born in Florence while her British parents were visiting Italy. Her parents were wealthy, and she and her sister were brought up on their father's estates in Derbyshire and Hampshire and received a classical education. It was assumed that she would take her place in polite society, and her announced intention to become a nurse was not favorably received. She took what opportunities occurred to nurse the sick in the villages near her home and was occasionally able to obtain hospital reports, which she studied carefully. In 1849, she went abroad with friends and visited a number of European hospitals.

In 1833, Theodore Fieldner, the pastor of a small German town, turned the garden house of his home into a training place for discharged female prisoners. With his wife's help, he trained these women to care for the sick, and in 1836, he founded the Institute of Protestant Deaconesses. In 1851, Florence Nightingale visited Kaiserwerth and trained in the Institute for three months. Subsequently, she spent some time at the Institute of St. Vincent de Paul in Paris before she returned to England. In 1853, she became lady superintendent of the Institute for Sick Gentlewomen in London.

Shortly after the outbreak of the Crimean War, in 1854, terrible reports of the British army hospital at Scutari, near Constantinople, caused grave concern in England, and Florence Nightingale wrote to her old friend Sidney Herbert, Secretary of State for War, offering her services. At precisely the same time, unaware that her letter was en route to him, Herbert wrote to her with the suggestion that she take over responsibility for all nursing activities associated with the Crimean War. In November 1854, she reached Scutari with about thirty nurses. The huge hospital was filthy and overcrowded; there was no proper drainage and no hot water; there were no medicines, beds, or bedding. Perhaps the most demoralizing thing was the inability of the doctors to make the government provide what was needed.

She had brought medical supplies and was well financed because of an appeal by *The Times,* so that the doctors, at first suspicious and disapproving, soon became her allies. In addition to organizing the whole hospital, including the repair and equipping of an entire wing, Florence Nightingale nursed the worst cases herself and was known to stay on the wards for more than twenty-four hours at a time. At night, she made her rounds with a lantern, and she is still remembered by the name given her by adoring soldiers, "The Lady with the Lamp."

In January 1855, there were twelve thousand men in Scutari and 42 percent of them died. By June, the death rate was only 2 percent. Later, Florence Nightingale traveled throughout the Crimea organizing and equipping hospitals, with similarly dramatic reductions in mortality rates.

When Florence Nightingale returned to England, she continued to work for improved nursing care and hygiene, particularly in the army, but would allow no public recognition of her remarkable services. However, in 1860, fifty thousand pounds, which had been collected in gratitude for her services in the Crimea, were used to found the Nightingale Training School for Nurses at St. Thomas' Hospital in London. In the same year, her *Notes on Nursing* was published; the first textbook for nurses, it was subsequently translated into many languages. The Nightingale School set high standards in discipline, behavior, and nursing skills so that Nightingale nurses were in great demand. In 1872, the New England Hospital for Women and Children in Boston offered a graded course in nursing, while the Bellevue Training School in New York, which was the first American school modeled on the Nightingale School, graduated its first class in 1875. In the course of a few years, nursing became established as an honorable profession.

Today, hospitals all over the world provide training programs for nurses, although in some places, especially in the United States, much of the education is college- rather than hospital-based. This trend has been slow to gain acceptance outside the United States. The development of nursing as a profession of dignity and esteem has been of incalculable benefit to sick people in all parts of the world.

8

Medicine in the Americas

AMONG PRIMITIVE societies, often widely separated in time and place, we have seen a basic pattern of response to illness that was divided into two parts. These were magico-religious medicine, the response to major illnesses occurring in the individual or in the group, particularly ill-understood conditions, such as mental illness, and empirical medicine that was employed in the cure or relief of day-to-day problems, such as disorders of the alimentary tract or rheumatism. Societies differed in the extent to which these were combined or separated and in the level of sophistication that had been achieved.

So it was with the indigenous population of North and South America. The available evidence indicates that their medical practices were remarkably similar to those of other primitive societies described earlier. Although the different life-styles of the nomadic, warring, northern Indians and the more settled farmers of the south were reflected in local medical practices, there was a generalized use of religious ceremonies, chants, and incantations based on a belief in the intervention of the gods (who would punish by inflicting illness) and in possession by demons. Surgery of war wounds was quite advanced, as was the use of herbal remedies.

As European settlers arrived, they brought their medical practices with them. The Spanish American countries naturally developed a system of medical education based on that of the mother country. Although the apprenticeship system was initially used to train physicians, licenses being granted by local examiners acting on behalf of the city councils as early as 1542, this system was modified. All medical matters, including medical education, were placed under the royal

155

protomedicate, as specified in the new laws of the Indies. Universities were established in Spanish America, and European medical graduates validated their diplomas in the new institutions before the establishment of chairs of medicine.

The first chair of medicine in the Americas was established in 1578 at the University of Mexico by Professor Juan de la Fuente (1530–95). By 1580, a regular four-year course for the degree of Bachelor of Medicine was approved. The curriculum was basically Galenic: First year, *de elementis*, parts of *de humeribus*, some anatomy, *de facultatibus naturalibus, de pulsibus ad tirenes;* second year, *de differentiis febrium, ars curativa ad Glauconem, de sanguinis missione;* third year, the aphorisms of Hippocrates, *quos et quando oportet purgari*, the ninth book of Rhazes' *ad Almansorem;* and fourth year, *de crisibus, de diebus decretoriis* and *de methodo medendi.*

Mexico was not, of course, the only Spanish American colony that had a medical school. In 1537, the city council of Lima, Peru, appointed a protomedicate to supervise medical education. For several years, students were licensed to practice medicine by Hernando Sepulveda, who had formerly taught at the University at Salamanca and had acted as personal physician to Francisco Pizarro. In 1551, the University of San Marcos was founded in Lima. The first degree of doctor of medicine conferred on American soil was granted in Peru in 1553.

During the colonial period, despite the numerous provisions for the training and licensing of physicians, the number of medical graduates was relatively small. On the average the University of Mexico granted from five to ten degrees per year; Peru, one to three; and Guatemala, one.

The University of Mexico was replaced by the Establishment of Medical Sciences in 1833. The vice-president of Mexico at that time, V. Gomez Farias (1781–1858), was a physician, and he was instrumental in founding the Establishment. The Establishment revolutionized medical education in Mexico with its fresh scientific approach. French clinical programs were incorporated with the texts, and students benefited from the expertise of such French medical scholars as J. P. Maygrier, F. Magendie, L. C. Roche, E. Tuortelle, and others. During the nineteenth century, the Establishment produced such outstanding clinicians as C. Liceaga, M. Carpio, M. Jimenez, R. Lucio, and I. Alvarado. The Medical School of Mexico had a five-year degree program and a School of Nursing and Obstetrics. The present Faculty of Medicine of the National University of Mexico is descended from the Establishment. In recent years, the School of Nursing and Obstetrics has become independent of the Medical School. By the close of the century, the Medical School had close to 400 students; by 1925, the School of Nursing and Obstetrics had graduated 381 nurses and 169 midwives. In 1965, there were 1,200 medical students per year graduating from the school.

In Peru, in 1807, J. Hipolito Unanue (1755–1833) requested that a medical school be established that was separate from the University of San Marcos. He had earlier initiated a program of weekly clinical lectures. The content of these lectures was surgery and internal medicine. In 1808, the Royal College of Medicine and Surgery of San Fernando was founded. Unanue proposed a curriculum that was based on the curricula of Paris and Leyden, including the following subjects: mathematics, physics, natural history, botany, anatomy, pathology, internal medicine, surgery, obstetrics, pharmacy, medical geography, drawing, languages, and field studies. When Peru became independent in 1821, the school became the College of the Independence. After 1826, when a hospital for clinical teaching was added, the college began to decline, and in 1850, it again became a part of the university. Cayetano Heredia (1797–1861), who was professor of anatomy from 1843 to 1856, was responsible for a number of reforms in Peruvian medical education.

Among the Latin American countries, Brazil has produced a number of notable men of medicine. Oswaldo Cruz (1872–1917) is regarded as one of the great pioneers in the field of public health. A student at the Pasteur Institute in Paris, he later returned to Rio de Janeiro, where he established the Oswaldo Cruz Institute (1908), which carried out important studies on plague, malaria, hematology, and serum therapy. Following Cruz's death in 1917, Carlos Chagas directed the institute and campaigned relentlessly against malaria, leprosy, and other diseases. Chagas is regarded as the discoverer of the mosquito vector of trypanosomiasis. The Oswaldo Cruz Institute now has its counterpart in most Latin American countries.

Unlike the Spanish, the English approach to colonization was more informal and relied upon private initiative. The Crown did not attempt to establish and finance colonies; this was left to companies and individuals who, although receiving a royal charter, were not official agents of the government. Thus, as it was not in keeping with royal policy to establish universities, as was the case with Spain, the first collegiate curriculum in medicine was not established in the English colonies until 1756.

University education, particularly medical education, developed after the colonial society in North America had matured.

Although the colonization of Virginia was carefully planned, the London Company neglected to provide adequately for the maintenance of the settlers' health. There was no physician sent with the first settlers. At this time, "physician" designated a practitioner with a university degree who specialized in teaching, studying, and/or the care of the upper classes. There was a gentleman-surgeon who served as physician to that first colonizing fleet, and one of the indentured servants was listed as a surgeon. English surgeons did not usually possess university degrees but were trained through apprenticeships and hospital instruction. Those who ministered to the ailing colonists usually served also as barbers; in many cases, the same razor that cut hair was used in the "surgical" process of bloodletting!

Although "barber-surgeons" were common in England (at this time the distinction between the two was negligible), the professions were apparently different in Virginia, as there is no record of any "barber-surgeon" in the colony. In any case, the early records of medical practice in the colony are very scant. Medical knowledge and practice in the colony must have been sadly deficient, for in the first summer more than half of the settlers died. This high mortality rate can be attributed in part to the lack of any consideration for public health in selecting the site for settlement. Although the London Company sent medical men to the colony (Lawrence Bohun, John Pott, and Robert Pawlett), there were few physicians in Virginia during the colonial period who were the products of the apprenticeship system, and prior to 1700, there were no more than four physicians in Virginia with medical degrees, in addition to a number of female nurses and midwives. At the time of the Revolution, there were only about four hundred men who held medical degrees in all the colonies—even though there were over thirty-five hundred physicians!

Medical practice in the New England colonies differed somewhat from that in Virginia. The earliest practitioner of medicine in the Plymouth colony, and in the whole of New England, was Deacon Samuel Fuller (1580–1633). Like most of the physicians of this region, he was also a minister, deacon of the church at Plymouth. Fuller was born in Norfolk County, England, and was educated as a theologian at the Dutch University of Leyden. Although Fuller undoubtedly absorbed some knowledge of medicine while studying at Leyden, he served as physician for the Plymouth colony for thirteen years without a medical degree.

Giles Firmin, Jr. (1615–97), was another man of the cloth who tended the ailing Puritans. Firmin is credited with being the first teacher of medicine in New England. He may have practiced in Boston in 1638; in the following year, he settled at Ipswich but returned to his native England in 1644. Other distinguished Puritans who were concerned with bodies as well as with souls were John Endicott, John Winthrop, and Cotton Mather. Mather (1663–1728) has been called the first significant figure in American medicine. In 1685, Mather, a graduate of Harvard, was ordained at the Second Church in Boston, where he remained for the rest of his life. Mather received his medical education from books; at the time of his matriculation, Harvard offered no courses in medicine.

It is probable that at Harvard Mather became familiar with the writings of Galen; Felix Plater, a sixteenth-century advocate of the practice of dissection; and Francis Le Boe, the seventeenth-century professor who introduced ward instruction into the curriculum of the University of Leyden. Although it is improbable that Mather ever practiced medicine in the strictest sense of the word, he did publish a treatise on measles in 1713 and gave his daughter Katy instruction in the preparation and dispensation of medicines. Although Mather would have preferred that the members of his flock receive care from competent and trained physicians, the practical side of his Puritan nature led him to urge clergymen to minister to the bodies of their congregations in the absence of genuine physicians. Between 1720 and 1724, he wrote *The Angel of Bethesda,* in which he argued that sinners could become physically diseased because of their moral and spiritual sickness. Hence, the physician-clergyman was the person best suited to cure illness. Mather was a forerunner of Christian Science and psychosomatic medicine.

As the ties between Great Britain and the colonies loosened, a university education was no longer a thing that could be obtained only in Europe. In 1636, Harvard was founded, followed in 1701 by Yale. Yet despite this advance in American education, at the time of the outbreak of the American Revolution, Philadelphia and New York were the only places where academic medical instruction was available. Almost all of those who wished to learn the practice of medicine received instruction from those relatively few physicians who, like Dr. William Shippen, Jr., of Philadelphia, had been educated in Europe. In 1781, the medical school of Harvard University was established; the medical school at Yale was not founded until 1810.

One of the most significant medical milestones of eighteenth-century America was the establishment of the Pennsylvania Hospital, in 1751. The two men responsible for the hospital were Dr. Thomas Bond (1712–84) and Benjamin Franklin. Bond had studied medicine in England, Scotland, and France. Although he recognized the need for an institution to care for the sick poor in Philadelphia, his efforts met with limited success until he introduced his idea to Benjamin Franklin, who suggested that they present the idea to the Pennsylvania Assembly. The "Act to encourage the establishing of an Hospital for the Relief of the Sick Poor of this province, and for the Reception and Cure of Lunaticks" was approved by the governor of Pennsylvania on May 11, 1751. The bill was initially jeopardized because members of the assembly were unwilling to incur the cost of such an establishment; the act was not passed until Thomas Bond and two other doctors, Lloyd Zachary and Phineas Bond, offered to donate their services. The hospital opened in February 1752, and fairly rigid standards were imposed on the staff; prospective members were required to have served an apprenticeship in Philadelphia or its suburbs and to have studied "physick and surgery" for at least seven years. The building that is still used today was completed in 1805.

Benjamin Franklin was not the only founding father to take an interest in the plight of the sick. Benjamin Rush (1744–1813), a signer of the Declaration of Independence and responsible for the renewal of friendship between Thomas Jefferson and John Adams after a long interval of silence, made many contributions to the medical profession. These include his achievements in the field of mental health. Rush's *Medical Inquiries and Observations upon the Diseases of the Mind,* published in 1812, was the first textbook dealing with the diseases of the mind by an American author. His observations were based upon practical experience; he had been in charge of mental patients at the Pennsylvania Hospital for thirty years. Rush was probably influenced by the work of Philippe Pinel, who was affiliated with the Paris School of Hygiene and who advocated a more humanitarian approach to the treatment of the mentally disturbed. Rush crusaded for the humane treatment of the insane because he believed that good health was ultimately the product of the individual's social, political, and economic environment as well as any physical factors that might be involved. In contrast to the earlier practitioners of medicine in America, he believed that the patient who suffered from mental illness should be treated with medicine rather than with moralizing. He felt that mental illness, like all illnesses, was a result of tension in the blood vessels. In the case of the insane, the blood vessels in the brain were abnormal, and the disease could be cured by bloodletting. Like other eighteenth-century physicians, Rush advocated the use of such practices as purging, cold showers, the stimulation of terror, and emetics —he was, at the time, one of the most humane physicians dealing with the problems of the mentally ill! Called the father of American psychiatry, Rush encouraged his patients to discuss their emotions with him and encouraged them on their way to recovery.

Dr. Samuel Bard (1716–99), a professor at the King's College School of Medicine, felt that the establishment of an institution for the care of the sick poor would benefit the entire community of New York. In 1769, the project was approved, but construction of the facility did not start until 1773. Unfortunately, the buildings were razed by fire before they were completed; this delayed the opening of the hospital until 1791. By the middle of the nineteenth century, the New York Hospital had earned a high reputation; operations requiring considerable skill and experience were performed there, and the doctors who served on the staff were reputed to be as competent as any European physicians of the day.

Although hospitals were important contributors to the public health of the colonies and of the young nation, the establishment of medical colleges was a significant and much-needed development. Dr. Shippen, mentioned above, and John Morgan (1735–89) were instrumental in the establishment of the School of Medicine of the University of Pennsylvania. Morgan arrived in Philadelphia in 1765 with a plan for a faculty of medicine for the College of Philadelphia, which had been founded in 1740. On May 3, 1765, he received approval for his plan, largely through the efforts of Thomas Penn, now the proprietor of the colony. He was appointed professor of Theory and Practice of Physic. Morgan felt that the establishment of a medical school was necessary because the traditional apprenticeship system was inadequate. He had heard of Shippen and his lectures on obstetrics and proposed establishing a chair of anatomy and surgery, which should be occupied by Shippen. Although the two professors could not offer a comprehensive course in medicine, they laid the foundations for what later became the University of Pennsylvania School of Medicine. The University Medical School was in turn the progenitor of a number of medical schools that were established during the first half of the nineteenth century.

Two years after the school in Philadelphia opened its doors, King's College in New York copied Morgan and Shippen's program. In 1769, ahead of its sister school, King's conferred its first advanced medical degree to Robert Tucker. During the revolution, the school closed down, and it reopened as Columbia College. Unfortunately, the medical school was not reopened. During this time, the void in medical education in New York was filled by such individual instructors as Dr. Nicholas Romayne (1756–1817). Romayne deplored the absence of institutionalized medical instruction, and in 1792, he was authorized to establish a College of Physicians and Surgeons. Columbia University, afraid that it would be eclipsed in the field of medical instruction, prevailed upon the regents of the University of New York to revoke Romayne's charter and issue a charter to Samuel Bard. Undaunted, Romayne founded the New York Medical Society in 1806, and in 1807, he got a charter to establish a College of Physicians and Surgeons, which in 1813 merged with the medical department at Columbia. Finally, in 1820, the college was reorganized and placed on a more solid foundation, which has enabled it to maintain its high standard until the present.

After the end of the Revolutionary War, settlers began to push through the mountains and to establish outposts in Kentucky, Tennessee, Ohio, Illinois, and Missouri. Just as trained and qualified doctors had been in short supply during colonization and revolution, there were not enough doctors in the western settlements to care for the eighteenth-century pioneers. In the 1730s, a Virginia scholar, John Tennent, published the manual *Every Man His Own Doctor*. Throughout the frontier area, self-appointed and self-trained physicians consulted this and similar publications in their efforts to provide medical and health care. Partially as a result of the scarcity of trained medical practitioners, the health standards of pioneer settlements were notoriously poor. The settler who was worn by hard labor suffered from the effects of improper diet. The nearby stream that furnished water was the home and breeding place of flies, gnats, and mosquitoes. The pioneers were completely unaware that malaria and other fevers that threatened their lives were spread by these pests. All too often frontier women relied on crude folk remedies, which included sweatings, chants, and some Indian methods. In 1813, Peter Smith (1753–1816), a self-taught physician, published *The Indian Doctor's Dispensary*, which enumerated frontier medical practices and dealt with Indian root and herb remedies. Those few men who did practice medicine in frontier settlements used methods that were at best crude. The many risks that the frontiersman faced frequently necessitated amputation. If the sufferer was fortunate enough to reach a doctor, a bottle of whisky and a crude set of amputating instruments removed the mangled limb. If not, he always had a knife with which to perform the necessary operation unassisted. In spite of the primitive conditions, several men added to medical experience and knowledge during the nineteenth century.

Daniel Drake (1785–1852) is often referred to as "the greatest physician of the West." At an early age, Drake moved with his family to Kentucky from New Jersey. Despite his fragmentary and haphazard early education, he received a medical degree from the University of Pennsylvania and was a renowned teacher and lecturer. In 1821, he founded the Medical College of Ohio, and in 1835, he established the Medical Department at Cincinnati College. *The Western Journal of Medical and Physical Sciences* (1827–38), the most important medical journal of the time, owed its existence to Drake. From 1850 to 1854, he wrote *Diseases of the Interior Valley of North America*. Drake was concerned that physicians who served the growing frontier society were inadequately educated. His advice was not generally taken when he recommended a four-year training period for physicians with practical bedside demonstrations.

During this period, Oliver Wendell Holmes (1809–94) practiced gynecology and made several important contributions to the field. Holmes was not only a poet and a man of letters; in February 1843, he read a paper before the Boston Society for Medical Improvement that discussed puerperal fever and the methods of its transmission. Upon presenting his paper, Holmes noted that, as the malady was contagious, physicians dealing with puerperal fever should not visit women who are confined in childbed. If this could not be avoided, the physician should be careful to wash his hands in calcium chloride and change clothes after leaving the patient with the fever. Although Holmes's views met with opposition in professional circles, he reiterated his thesis in 1855, when he published *Puerperal Fever as a Private Pestilence*. Here is the concluding statement from the paper:

In connection with the facts which have been stated it seems proper to allude to the dangerous and often fatal effects which have followed from wounds received in the post-mortem examination of patients who have died of puerperal fever. The fact that such wounds are attended with peculiar risk has been long noticed. I find that Chaussier was in the habit of cautioning his students against the danger to which they were exposed in these dissections. The head *pharmacien* of the Hôtel Dieu, in his analysis of the fluid effused in puerperal peritonitis, says that practitioners are convinced of its deleterious qualities, and that it is very dangerous to apply it to the denuded skin. Sir Benjamin Brodie speaks of it as being well known that the inoculation of lymph or pus from the peritoneum of a puerperal patient is often attended with dangerous and even fatal symptoms. Three cases in confirmation of this statement, two of them fatal, have been reported to this society within a few months.

Of about fifty cases of injuries of this kind, of various degrees of severity, which I have collected from different sources, at least twelve were instances of infection from puerperal peritonitis. Some of the others are so stated as to render it probable that they may have been of the same nature. Five other cases were of peritoneal inflammation; three in males. Three were what was called enteritis, in one instance complicated with erysipelas; but it is well known that this term has been often used to signify inflammation of the peritoneum covering the intestines. On the other hand, no case of typhus or typhoid fever is mentioned as giving rise to dangerous consequences, with the exception of the single instance of an undertaker mentioned by Mr. Travers, who seems to have been poisoned by a fluid which exuded from the body. The other accidents were produced by dissection, or some other mode of contact with bodies of patients who had died of various affections. They also differed much in severity, the cases of puerperal origin being among the most formidable and fatal. Now a moment's reflection will show that the number of cases of serious consequences ensuing from the dissection of the bodies of those who had perished of puerperal fever is so vastly disproportioned to the relatively small number of autopsies made in this complaint as compared with typhus or pneumonia (from which last disease not one case of poisoning happened) and still more from all diseases put together that the conclusion is irresistible that a most fearful morbid poison is often generated in the course of this disease. Whether or not it is *sui generis* confined to this disease, or produced in some others, as, for instance, erysipelas, I need not stop to inquire.

In connection with this may be taken the following statement of Dr. Rigby: "That the discharges from a patient under puerperal fever are in the highest degree contagious we have abundant evidence in the history of lying-in hospitals. The puerperal abscesses are also contagious, and may be communicated to healthy lying-in women by washing with the same sponge; this fact has been repeatedly proved in the Vienna Hospital; but they are equally communicable to women not pregnant; on more than one occasion the women engaged "in washing the soiled bed-linen of the General Lying-in Hospital have been attacked with abscesses in the fingers or hands, attended with rapidly spreading inflammation of the cellular tissue."

Now add to all this the undisputed fact that within the walls of lying-in hospitals there is often generated a miasm, palpable as the chlorine used to destroy it, tenacious so as in some cases almost to defy extirpation, deadly in some institutions as the plague; which has killed women in a private hospital of London so fast that they were buried two in one coffin to conceal its horrors; which enabled Tonnellé to record two hundred and twenty-two autopsies at the Maternité of Paris; which has led Dr. Lee to express his deliberate conviction that the loss of life occasioned by these institutions completely defeats the objects of their founders; and out of this train of cumulative evidence, the multiplied groups of cases clustering about individuals, the deadly results of autopsies, the inoculation by fluids from the living patient, the murderous poison of hospitals—does there not result a conclusion that laughs all sophistry to scorn, and renders all argument an insult?

I have had occasion to mention some instances in which there was an apparent relation between puerperal fever and erysipelas. The length to which this paper has extended does not allow me to enter into the consideration of this most important subject. I will only say that the evidence appears to me altogether satisfactory that some most fatal series of puerperal fever have been produced by an infection originating in the matter or effluvia of erysipelas. In evidence of some connection between the two diseases, I need not go back to the older authors, as Pouteau or Gordon, but will content myself with giving the following references, with their dates; from which it will be seen that the testimony has been constantly coming before the profession for the last few years:

"London Cyclopaedia of Practical Medicine," article Puerperal Fever, 1833.

Mr. Ceeley's Account of the Puerperal Fever at Aylesbury, "Lancet," 1835.

Dr. Ramsbotham's Lecture, "London Medical Gazette," 1835.

Mr. Yates Ackerly's Letter in the same journal, 1838.

Mr. Ingleby on Epidemic Puerperal Fever, "Edinburgh Medical and Surgical Journal," 1838.

Mr. Paley's Letter, "London Medical Gazette," 1839.

Remarks at the Medical and Chirurgical Society, "Lancet," 1840.

Dr. Rigby's "System of Midwifery," 1841.

"Nunneley on Erysipelas," a work which contains a large number of references on the subject, 1841.

"British and Foreign Quarterly Review," 1842.

Dr. S. Jackson, of Northumberland, as already quoted from the Summary of the College of Physicians, 1842.

And, lastly, a startling series of cases by Mr. Storrs, of Doncaster, to be found in the "American Journal of the Medical Sciences" for January, 1843.

The relation of puerperal fever with other continued fevers would seem to be remote and rarely obvious. Hey refers to two cases of synochus occurring in the Royal Infirmary of Edinburgh, in women who had attended upon puerperal patients. Dr. Collins refers to several instances in which puerperal fever has appeared to originate from a continued proximity to patients suffering with typhus.

Such occurrences as those just mentioned, though most important to be remembered and guarded against, hardly attract our notice in the midst of the gloomy facts by which they are surrounded. Of these facts, at the risk of fatiguing repetitions, I have summoned a sufficient number, as I believe, to convince the most incredulous that every attempt to disguise the truth which underlies them all is useless.

It is true that some of the historians of the disease, especially Hulme, Hull, and Leake, in England; Tonnellé, Dugès, and Baudelocque, in France, profess not to have found puerperal fever contagious. At the most they give us mere negative facts, worthless against an extent of evidence which now overlaps the widest range of doubt, and doubles upon itself in the redundancy of superfluous demonstration. Examined in detail, this and much of the show of testimony brought up to stare the daylight of conviction out of countenance, proves to be in a great measure unmeaning and inapplicable, as might be easily shown were it necessary. Nor do I feel the necessity of enforcing the conclusion which arises spontaneously from the facts which have been enumerated by formally citing the opinions of those grave authorities who have for the last half-century been sounding the unwelcome truth it has cost so many lives to establish.

"It is to the British practitioner," says Dr. Rigby, "that we are indebted for strongly insisting upon this important and dangerous character of puerperal fever."

The names of Gordon, John Clarke, Denman, Burns, Young, Hamilton,

Haighton, Good, Waller, Blundell, Gooch, Ramsbotham, Douglas, Lee, Ingleby, Locock, Abercrombie, Alison, Travers, Rigby, and Watson many of whose writings I have already referred to, may have some influence with those who prefer the weight of authorities to the simple deductions of their own reason from the facts laid before them. A few Continental writers have adopted similar conclusions. It gives me pleasure to remember that, while the doctrine has been unceremoniously discredited in one of the leading journals, and made very light of by teachers in two of the principal medical schools of this country, Dr. Channing has for many years inculcated, and enforced by examples, the danger to be apprehended and the precautions to be taken in the disease under consideration.

I have no wish to express any harsh feeling with regard to the painful subject which has come before us. If there are any so far excited by the story of these dreadful events that they ask for some word of indignant remonstrance to show that science does not turn the hearts of its followers into ice or stone, let me remind them that such words have been uttered by those who speak with an authority I could not claim. It is as a lesson rather than as a reproach that I call up the memory of these irreparable errors and wrongs. No tongue can tell the heart-breaking calamity they have caused; they have closed the eyes just opened upon a new world of love and happiness; they have bowed the strength of manhood into the dust; they have cast the helplessness of infancy into the stranger's arms, or bequeathed it, with less cruelty, the death of its dying parent. There is no tone deep enough for regret, and no voice loud enough for warning. The woman about to become a mother or with her newborn infant upon her bosom, should be the object of trembling care and sympathy wherever she bears her tender burden or stretches her aching limbs. The very outcast of the streets has pity upon her sister in degradation when the seal of promised maternity is impressed upon her. The remorseless vengeance of the law, brought down upon its victim by a machinery as sure as destiny, is arrested in its fall at a word which reveals her transient claim for mercy. The solemn prayer of the liturgy singles out her sorrows from the multiplied trials of life, to plead for her in the hour of peril. God forbid that any member of the profession to which she trusts her life, doubly precious at that eventful period, should hazard it negligently, unadvisedly, or selfishly!

There may be some among those whom I address who are disposed to ask the question, What course are we to follow in relation to this matter? The facts are before them, and the answer must be left to their own judgment and conscience. If any should care to know my own conclusions, they are the following; and in taking the liberty to state them very freely and broadly, I would ask the inquirer to examine them as freely in the light of the evidence which has been laid before him.

1. A physician holding himself in readiness to attend cases of midwifery

should never take any active part in the post-mortem examination of cases of puerperal fever.

2. If a physician is present at such autopsies, he should use thorough ablution, change every article of dress, and allow twenty-four hours or more to elapse before attending to any case of midwifery. It may be well to extend the same caution to cases of simple peritonitis.

3. Similar precautions should be taken after the autopsy or surgical treatment of cases of erysipelas, if the physician is obliged to unite such offices with his obstetrical duties, which is in the highest degree inexpedient.

4. On the occurrence of a single case of puerperal fever in his practice, the physician is bound to consider the next female he attends in labor, unless some weeks at least have elapsed, as in danger of being infected by him, and it is his duty to take every precaution to diminish her risk of disease and death.

5. If within a short period two cases of puerperal fever happen close to each other, in the practice of the same physician, the disease not existing or prevailing in the neighborhood, he would do wisely to relinquish his obstetrical practice for at least one month, and endeavor to free himself by every available means from any noxious influence he may carry about with him.

6. The occurrence of three or more closely connected cases, in the practice of one individual, no others existing in the neighborhood, and no other sufficient cause being alleged for the coincidence, is *prima facie* evidence that he is the vehicle of contagion.

7. It is the duty of the physician to take every precaution that the disease shall not be introduced by nurses or other assistants, by making proper inquiries concerning them, and giving timely warning of every suspected source of danger.

8. Whatever indulgence may be granted to those who have heretofore been the ignorant causes of so much misery, the time has come when the existence of a *private pestilence* in the sphere of a single physician should be looked upon, not as a misfortune, but a crime; and in the knowledge of such occurrences the duties of the practitioner to his profession should give way to his paramount obligations to society.

Another important nineteenth century physician, James Marion Sims (1813–83), is considered to be the founder of gynecology in the United States. The South Carolina native made a useful contribution to the profession when he conducted a successful operation for vaginal fistula in 1849. After his graduation from Jefferson Medical College, in 1835, Sims embarked on a brilliant career. In 1852, he published a paper in the *American Journal of Medical Sciences* that described several of his cures for vesicovaginal fistulas, which until that time had not been treated successfully. When he moved to New York in 1853, Sims established the State Hospital for Women, which was noted for the best gynecological care in the country. In 1861, Sims developed a method for removing the uterine neck by surgery, and in 1878, he developed an operation for disease of the gallbladder.

Sims was one of the first American physicians to receive recognition in Europe, and in the following selection, he recounts some of his experiences in Paris and the hazards of chloroform anesthesia:

I had now performed four operations, in four of the most prominent hospitals in Paris, and before all the leading surgeons of the city, and my work was the theme of conversation among medical men everywhere. Men attending the hospitals wrote to different parts of the world, even to Russia and back to my own country, about the work that I was doing in Paris.

Very soon after the operation for Velpeau, in La Charité Hospital, Dr. Mungenier, who had taken a great interest in me and my work, and who, with Dr. Johnstone had been prominent in introducing me to the surgeons of hospitals, brought me a woman about forty years old who had had a vesico-vaginal fistula for more than twenty years. She had been seen and examined by many of the leading surgeons of Paris, and pronounced incurable. She had also been seen by the American surgeon who preceded me in Paris three years previously, and who had refused to operate upon her. The case was certainly a very bad one. The whole base of the bladder was destroyed, the mouths of the ureters were plainly visible, and the urine could be seen passing in little spurts from these narrow openings. The bladder was inverted and hung outside of the body, in a little hernial mass as large as a child's fist. Her condition was very deplorable, and my friend Dr. Mungenier was very much surprised when I told him she could easily be cured by a single operation. He said, "But I can't get a bed for her in any hospital." I replied, "That makes no difference; I will take her to the Hôtel Voltaire and engage a room and will pay the expenses myself, just to show you that I can cure her."

He was very much surprised that I should be willing to do this, and then he said, "I can bring many of the leading surgeons from the different hospitals to see you operate if you will let me." I agreed to it, and the operation was performed at the Hôtel Voltaire on the 18th of October, 1861. I was greatly surprised to see that a number of leading physicians were not only willing, but anxious, to witness the operation in private practice. Among them were Nélaton, Velpeau, Civiale, Baron Larrey, Sir Joseph Olliffe, Campbell, Huguier, and others of the most distinguished men of Paris, numbering to about seventeen or eighteen. Dr. Johnstone gave the anaesthetic. The operation required about an hour; the fistula was closed to the satisfaction of everybody present. In one week's time the sutures, twelve in number, were removed and the patient was found perfectly cured.

As a matter of course, these five successful operations in three or four weeks in the great city of Paris, created a *furore* among the profession in regard to the curability of an affection which they had until now supposed to be totally incurable.

Having thus demonstrated clearly the principles and success of the operation in the hospitals of Paris, I was on the eve of going to Vienna to do something in that city, when Dr. Campbell, the great *accoucheur* of Paris, told Dr. Nélaton that I was about to leave. Dr. Nélaton asked Dr. Campbell to see me and beg me to remain for a few days, till he could go for a patient to come to me from the south of France. The patient had been seen six or eight months previous, and pronounced perfectly incurable. "But," said he to Dr. Campbell, "since I have witnessed what I have in the hands of Dr. Sims, and since I have heard of the success attending his operations in other hospitals, I think that he can cure almost any case of the sort. I am anxious to get his opinion in the case of this lady, who belongs to the higher walks of life." Of course I was too good a tactician to let such an opportunity as this pass without improving it, and I immediately sent word that I would await the arrival of his patient from the country. I did not get to Vienna at all, as a consequence.

His patient arrived in due time. She was about twenty-one. She had been delivered two years before. The child had *hydrocephalus,* the pressure of its enormous head produced a sloughing of the soft parts of the mother, which resulted in, seemingly, a total destruction of the base of the bladder. She was young, beautiful, rich, accomplished; and, as Dr. Nélaton had told her six months before that she was absolutely incurable, she was praying for death, but in vain, for patients seldom die of afflictions of this kind. In all my experience I have never seen a case of this kind which was attended with such extreme suffering. The constant discharge of the urine had created an inflammation and excoriation of the external parts with which it came in contact, in some places producing sloughings as large as a pea. It looked like localized small-pox. She was obliged to take anodynes in large quantities to relieve the burning pain attendant upon her sufferings. She passed sleepless nights and restless days, and was altogether one of the most unhappy women I have ever seen.

On examination of the case I saw that it was exceedingly difficult. At first I was almost disposed to say it was incurable, but after a more thorough investigation I said to Dr. Nélaton that I was sure she could be cured; that it would require a little preparatory operation which would take a week or ten days, and the radical operation would be performed afterward, and I was convinced she could be restored perfectly. I went on to explain to him how the operation was to be done, thinking as a matter of course that he simply wanted my opinion on the question. He heard me patiently and said, "I understand everything that you say, but I don't feel competent to do the work. I have not the experience nor the skill of manipulation that you possess, and, if you will kindly take charge of my patient and perform this operation in my stead, I shall be greatly obliged to you." As a matter of course I accepted the case, which prevented me from making my proposed visit to Vienna.

The first operation, as I had indicated to Dr. Nélaton, was performed in the country, and in two weeks afterward the radical operation was performed at St. Germain, an hour's distance from Paris. Dr. Nélaton, Dr. Johnstone, Dr. Campbell, Dr. Beylard and Dr. Alan Herbert were my assistants.

Dr. Campbell was the great *accoucheur* of Paris at that time. He was in the habit of giving chloroform to his patients in labor, and was selected by the family to give the chloroform because of his known reputation in using it. The operation was begun at ten o'clock in the morning of the 19th of December, 1861, Dr. Nélaton sitting by and watching every stage of it with the greatest attention. At the end of about forty minutes all the sutures were introduced and ready to be secured. Just at this time I discovered a certain amount of lividity in the mucous surfaces, and I called Dr. Nélaton's and Dr. Johnstone's attention to it, and said, "It seems to me the blood is stagnating." I asked Dr. Campbell if the pulse and respiration were all right; he said, "Yes, all right; go on." Scarcely were these words uttered when he suddenly cried out, "Stop! Stop! No pulse, no breathing." And sure enough the patient looked as if she was dead. Dr. Nélaton was not in the least disconcerted. He quietly ordered the head to be lowered and the body to be inverted, that is, the head to hang down while the heels were raised in the air by Dr. Johnstone, the legs resting one on each of his shoulders. Dr. Campbell supported the thorax, Dr. Herbert went to an adjoining room for a spoon with the handle of which the jaws were forced open, and I handed Dr. Nélaton the tenaculum, which he hooked in the tongue, pulling it out between the teeth, and gave it in charge of Dr. Herbert, while Dr. Beylard was assigned to the duty of making efforts at artificial respiration. Dr. Nélaton ordered and overlooked every movement. They held the patient in this inverted position for a long time, making artificial respiration, before there was any manifestation of returning life. Dr. Campbell, who published an account of the case subsequently, said in his report that it was fifteen minutes, and that it seemed an age. My notes of the case, written a few hours afterward, make it twenty minutes that the patient was held in this position. Be this as it may, the time was so long that I thought it useless to make any further efforts, and I said,

"Dr. Nélaton, our patient is dead, and you might as well stop all efforts."
But Dr. Nélaton never lost hope, and by his quiet, cool, brave manner he
seemed to infuse his spirit into his assistants. At last there was a feeble
inspiration, and after a long time another, and by and by another; and then
the breathing became regular. When the pulse and respiration were well
re-established, Dr. Nélaton ordered the patient to be laid on the table. This
was done very gently, but the moment the body was placed horizontally the
pulse and breathing instantly ceased. Quick as thought the body was again
inverted, the head downward and the feet over Dr. Johnstone's shoulders,
and the same manoeuvres as before were put into execution. Dr. Campbell
thinks it did not take such a long time to re-establish the action of the lungs
and heart as in the first instance, but it seemed to me to be quite as long, for
the same painful, protracted and anxious efforts were made as before. Feeble
signs of returning life eventually made their appearance. Respiration was at
first irregular and at long intervals; soon it became more regular, and the
pulse could then be counted, but it was very feeble and intermittent. When
they thought she had quite recovered they laid her horizontally on the table
again, saying "She's all right this time."

But the moment the body was placed in a horizontal position the respiration ceased a third time, the pulse was gone, and she looked the picture of
death. But Dr. Nélaton and his assistants, by a simultaneous effort, quickly
inverted the body a third time, with a view of throwing all the blood possible
to the brain, and again they began their efforts at artificial respiration. It
seemed to me that she would never breathe again, but at last there was a
spasmodic gasp, and after a long time another, and after another long interval
there was a third, and then a fourth more profoundly; there was then a long
yawn, and the respiration after this became tolerably regular. She was held
in a vertical position until she in a manner became semi-conscious, opened
her eyes, looked wildly around, and asked what was the matter. She was then,
and not until then, laid on the table, and we all thanked Dr. Nélaton for
having saved the life of this lovely woman. In a few minutes more the
operation was finished, but of course without any more chloroform. The
sutures were quickly assorted and separately secured, and the patient put to
bed. On the eighth day thereafter I had the happiness to remove the sutures,
in the presence of Dr. Nélaton, and to show him the success of the operation.

Although Sir Humphry Davy had suggested the possibility of using
ether and nitrous oxide as anesthetics as early as 1800, it was nearly
half a century before the potential value of these gases was recognized.
In 1844, a Connecticut dentist, Horace Wells (1815–47), began to
use nitrous oxide to anesthetize his patients, and a colleague, William

Thomas Green Morton (1819–68), aware of Wells's success, employed ether anesthesia in his dental practice. Morton subsequently approached a prominent Boston surgeon, John Collins Warren, with the suggestion of a trial of ether anesthesia in a surgical operation. The trial operation took place on October 16, 1846, at the Massachusetts General Hospital with complete success.

During the Civil War, great strides were made in the field of surgical procedure, aided by the use of surgical anesthesia, which became more and more common as military surgeons sought to repair the many casualties of this bloody conflict. In 1862, William Alexander Hammond was appointed Surgeon General of the Army. Hammond insisted that accurate records of casualties and camp diseases be kept and that better and more detailed reports of all treatments be filed. This large body of information later proved useful as doctors sought to improve medical practice.

John Shaw Billings (1838–1913), like many of the physicians of his day, served as an army surgeon during the Civil War. He practiced both in hospitals and at the front and was present at the battle of Gettysburg. In 1860, he graduated from the Medical College of Ohio. Billings was particularly sensitive to the lack of library facilities, especially to the shortage of medical texts. It was his desire for knowledge combined with his need for books, that led him to be called the father of the American medical library. In 1864, he was appointed surgeon general, and recognizing that the medical library in Washington was deficient, he began to build a national library of medicine around the 1,365 volumes that he found there. As Surgeon General, he secured federal funds to underwrite the project, and by 1876, the library had forty thousand volumes. With the aid of Robert Fletcher and Fielding H. Garrison, Billings produced an index catalogue that is still of value to medical investigators. Thirty years after his appointment as Surgeon General, Billings left that post and served as Visiting Professor of Hygiene at the University of Pennsylvania. Shortly thereafter he became the director of the New York Public Library. The present quarters of the library on Fifth Avenue were built according to his plans. As Surgeon General, Billings also undertook to reorganize the Marine Hospital Service. This agency was responsible for quarantining harbors and for the health of the sailors in the merchant marine. Billings greatly reformed the agency, which in 1912 became the United States Public Health Service. An authority on hospitals, Billings was consulted by the builders of Johns Hopkins Hospital in Baltimore, which was initiated in 1876. Included among his numerous contributions to the medical profession were his achievements in the area of vital statistics. As a result of his efforts, the 1880 census of the American population included medical data.

One of the most well known physicians of the early twentieth century was Canadian-born William Osler (1849–1919), who came to the United States in 1884 to serve as professor of clinical medicine at the University of Pennsylvania. In 1889, he was asked to be a member of the medical faculty of Johns Hopkins, where he remained until he went to Oxford in 1905. Osler did a great deal of work in the field of pathological anatomy and was one of the first to study blood platelets. Under his direction, and largely due to the force of his engaging and warm personality, the clinic at Johns Hopkins became a center of scientific life and investigation. As a medical school, Johns Hopkins became noted for its emphasis on science, with the students sharing in the research and receiving instruction in the laboratory and in the wards. Throughout his career, Osler followed the scientific approach, and is remembered by physicians to this day for his humanitarianism. He was given a baronetcy in 1911 in recognition of his outstanding abilities. Typical of his writing is the following selection from *Aequanimitas,* an address to a graduating medical class:

In the second place, there is a mental equivalent to this bodily endowment, which is as important in our pilgrimage as imperturbability. Let me recall to your minds an incident related of that best of men and wisest of rulers, Antonius Pius, who, as he lay dying, in his home at Lorium in Etruria, summed up the philosophy of life in the watch word, *Aequanimitas.* As for him, about to pass *flammantia moenia mundi* (the flaming ramparts of the world), so for you, fresh from Clotho's spindle, a calm equanimity is the desirable attitude. How difficult to attain, yet how necessary, in success as in failure! Natural temperament has much to do with its development, but a clear knowledge of our relation to our fellow-creatures and to the work of life is also indispensable. One of the first essentials in securing a good-natured equanimity is not to expect too much of the people amongst whom you dwell. "Knowledge comes, but wisdom lingers," and in matters medical the ordinary citizen of to-day has not one whit more sense than the old Romans, whom Lucian scourged for a credulity which made them fall easy victims to the quacks of the time, such as the notorious Alexander, whose exploits make one wish that his advent had been delayed some eighteen centuries. Deal gently then with this deliciously credulous old human nature in which we work, and restrain your indignation, when you find your pet parson has triturates of the 1000th potentiality in his waistcoat pocket, or you discover accidentally a case of Warner's Safe Cure in the bedroom of your best patient. It must needs be that offences of this kind come; expect them, and do not be vexed.

Curious, odd compounds are these fellow-creatures, at whose mercy you will be; full of fads and eccentricities, of whims and fancies; but the more closely we study their little foibles of one sort and another in the inner life which we see, the more surely is the conviction borne in upon us of the likeness of their weaknesses to our own. The similarity would be intolerable, if a happy egotism did not often render us forgetful of it. Hence the need of an infinite patience and of an ever-tender charity toward these fellow-creatures; have they not to exercise the same toward us?

A distressing feature in the life which you are about to enter, a feature which will press hardly upon the finer spirits among you and ruffle their equanimity, is the uncertainty which pertains not alone to our science and art, but to the very hopes and fears which make us men. In seeking absolute truth we aim at the unattainable, and must be content with finding broken portions. You remember in the Egyptian story, how Typhon with his conspirators dealt with good Osiris; how they took the virgin Truth, hewed her lovely form into a thousand pieces, and scattered them to the four winds; and, as Milton says, "from that time ever since, the sad friends of truth, such as durst appear, imitating the careful search that Isis made for the mangled body of Osiris, went up and down gathering up limb by limb still as they could find them. We have not yet found them all," but each one of us may pick up a fragment, perhaps two, and in moments when mortality weighs less heavily upon the spirit, we can, as in a vision, see the form divine, just as a great Naturalist, an Owen or a Leidy, can reconstruct an ideal creature from a fossil fragment.

It has been said that in prosperity our equanimity is chiefly exercised in enabling us to bear with composure the misfortunes of our neighbours. Now, while nothing disturbs our mental placidity more sadly than straitened means, and the lack of those things after which the Gentiles seek, I would warn you against the trials of the day soon to come to some of you—the day of large and successful practice. Engrossed late and soon in professional cares, getting and spending, you may so lay waste your powers that you may find, too late, with hearts given away, that there is no place in your habit-stricken souls for those gentler influences which make life worth living.

It is sad to think that, for some of you, there is in store disappointment, perhaps failure. You cannot hope, of course, to escape from the cares and anxieties incident to professional life. Stand up bravely, even against the worst. Your very hopes may have passed on out of sight, as did all that was near and dear to the Patriarch at the Jabbok ford, and, like him, you may be left to struggle in the night alone. Well for you, if you wrestle on, for in persistency lies victory, and with the morning may come the wished for blessing. But not always; there is a struggle with defeat which some of you will have to bear, and it will be well for you in that day to have cultivated a cheerful equanimity. Remember, too, that sometimes "from our desolation only does the better life begin." Even with disaster ahead and ruin imminent, it is better to face them with a smile, and with the head erect, than to crouch at their approach. And, if the fight is for principle and justice, even when failure seems certain, where many have failed before, cling to your ideal, and, like Childe Roland before the dark tower, set the slug-horn to your lips, blow the challenge, and calmly await the conflict.

As in other countries, the late nineteenth century saw in America the rise of medical specialization. The American Ophthalmological Society was founded in New York in 1864, and the American Otological Society was founded in 1868. The precursor of the American Psychiatric Society was also in existence at this time.

The second half of the nineteenth century saw the growth of the sectarian approach to medical treatment. Seen as quacks by the regular practitioners, the founders of these medical sects produced their own medical schools and medical journals. Thomsonianism, a sect that advocated treatment by "steaming" and the extensive use of botanicals, was founded by Samuel Thomson (1769–1843) and was patented as early as 1813. The Botanico-Medical College of Ohio in Cincinnati was chartered in 1838, and the following year, the Southern Botanico-Medical College was established. In 1825, the practice of homeopathy was introduced in the United States. Osteopathy originated in the United States in 1874. The sectarians believed that ultimately there was one universal cause of disease; it followed logically, that there was one cure for disease.

The early twentieth century witnessed in the United States a movement to reform medical education and medical schools. Instrumental in this reform was Abraham Flexner (1866–1959), who in 1908 was assigned the task of evaluating medical education by the trustees of the Carnegie Foundation for the Advancement of Teaching. Flexner was a noted authority in the field of education at the time. He exposed the dreadful conditions in many of the contemporary medical schools, but the Flexner report was most significant because it offered constructive suggestions for the improvement of medical schools and medical education. The Association of American Medical Colleges had been formed in 1876, and after a period of inactivity, it was reestablished in 1890. Although there were a great many medical schools in the country at this time, few maintained desirable standards. Starting in 1807 with the establishment of a medical school by the Medical Society of the County of New York, society-affiliated institutions, called "proprietary" medical colleges, were started throughout the country. They were able to attract students because they did not require long general educations or long lecture terms. Not surprisingly, these institutions failed to train adequately these prospective doctors. The nineteenth century had seen the rapid growth of institutions for medical education. Sixty-two medical schools were established between 1802 and 1876, in addition to eleven homeopathic and four eclectic schools. Still, quality medical education was difficult to obtain; quality was sacrificed in order to increase the number of medical schools and medical graduates.

Flexner, alarmed at this situation, believed that quality medical education could only be obtained by reducing the number and by improving the quality of medical schools. He advocated that medical schools be university departments and ideally be located in large cities, where there would be no problem in procuring clinical material. Flexner noted that students tended to study medicine in their native states; hence, it was imperative that medical schools throughout the nation offer similar courses of instruction that are of uniform quality. The topic of varying standards is addressed quite early in his 1910 report to the Carnegie Foundation, *Medical Education in the United States and Canada:*

THE PROPER BASIS OF MEDICAL EDUCATION

We have in the preceding chapter briefly indicated three stages in the development of medical education in America,—the preceptorship, the didactic school, the scientific discipline. We have seen how an empirical training of varying excellence, secured through attendance on a preceptor, gave way to the didactic method, which simply communicated a set body of doctrines of very uneven value; how in our own day this didactic school has capitulated to a procedure that seeks, as far as may be, to escape empiricism in order to base the practice of medicine on observed facts of the same order and cogency as pass muster in other fields of pure and applied science. The apprentice saw disease; the didactic pupil heard and read about it; now once more the medical student returns to the patient, whom in the main he left when he parted with his preceptor. But he returns, relying no longer altogether on the senses with which nature endowed him, but with those senses made infinitely more acute, more accurate, and more helpful by the processes and the instruments which the last half-century's progress has placed at his disposal. This is the meaning of the altered aspect of medical training: the old preceptor, be he never so able, could at best feel, see, smell, listen, with his unaided senses. His achievements are not indeed to be lightly dismissed; for his sole reliance upon his senses greatly augmented their power. Succeed as he might however, his possibilities in the way of reducing, differentiating, and interpreting phenomena, or significant aspects of phenomena, were abruptly limited by his natural powers. These powers are nowadays easily enough transcended. The self-registering thermometer, the stethoscope, the microscope, the correlation of observed symptoms with the outgivings of chemical analysis and biological experimentation, enormously extend the physician's range. He perceives more speedily and more accurately what he is actually dealing with; he knows with far greater assurance the merits or the limitations of the agents which he is in position to invoke. Though the field of knowledge and certainty is even yet far from coextensive with the field of disease and injury, it is, as far as it goes, open to quick, intelligent, and effective action.

Provided, of course, the physician is himself competent to use the instrumentalities that have been developed! There is just now the rub. Society reaps at this moment but a small fraction of the advantage which current knowledge has the power to confer. That sick man is relatively rare for whom actually all is done that is at this day humanly feasible,—as feasible in the small hamlet as in the large city, in the public hospital as in the private sanatorium. We have indeed in America medical practitioners not inferior to the best elsewhere; but there is probably no other country in the world in which there is so great a distance and so fatal a difference between the best, the average, and the worst.

He also advocated an adequate preparation for entry to medical school:

From the foregoing discussion, these conclusions emerge: By the very nature of the case, admission to a really modern medical school must at the very least depend on a competent knowledge of chemistry, biology, and physics. Every departure from this basis is at the expense of medical training itself. From the exclusive standpoint of the medical school it is immaterial where the student gets the instruction. But it is clear that if it is to become the common minimum basis of medical education, some recognized and organized manner of obtaining it must be devised: it cannot be left to the initiative of the individual without greatly impairing its quality. Regular provision must therefore be made at a definite moment of normal educational progress. Now the requirement above agreed on is too extensive and too difficult to be incorporated in its entirety within the high school or to be substituted for a considerable portion of the usual high school course; besides, it demands greater maturity than the secondary school student can be credited with except towards the close of his high school career. The possibility of mastering the three sciences outside of school may be dismissed without argument. In the college or technical school alone can the work be regularly, efficiently, and surely arranged for. The requirement is therefore necessarily a college requirement, covering two years, because three laboratory courses cannot be carried through in a briefer period,—a fortunate circumstance, since it favors the student's simultaneous development along other and more general lines. It appears, then, that a policy that at the outset was considered from the narrow standpoint of the medical school alone shortly involves the abandonment of this point of view in favor of something more comprehensive. The preliminary requirement for entrance upon medical education must therefore be formulated in terms that establish a distinct relation, pedagogical and chronological, between the medical school and other educational agencies. Nothing will do more to steady and to improve the college itself than its assumption of such definite functions in respect to professional and other forms of special training.

In a further report to the Carnegie Foundation in 1912, *Medical Education in Europe,* Flexner points out the need for a close relationship between teaching and research and sets Germany before us as the leader in this field:

Vitality of advanced teaching requires the proximity of investigation; and the fields open to investigation are too rich and too extensive to be completely occupied by institutions of a single type. Occasional geniuses of peculiar intensity may be set aside in research establishments solely for productive work; the more common but not less useful type of scientist may find uninterrupted application to either teaching or research insupportable. A modicum of routine in the shape of teaching may then assist research, just as research will help to illuminate one's teaching. The same holds also of industrial or other practical activities. Factories, health offices, and other establishments of similar character have their own routine; but routine itself is most intelligent if those ultimately responsible for its direction promote fundamental study of the problems which it involves or suggests. There are better ways to do what is being done; there are better things to do. Hence a really effective organization will never limit itself to routine. The marvelous progress of German industry, German sanitation, German hospitals, is due in no small measure to the fact that industry, sanitation, and medical care have, like university teaching, cultivated research in all relevant directions. Institutes for pure research will, then, to some extent be established and liberally sustained. But research will still continue to animate university laboratories, municipal hospitals, industrial establishments, and sanitary institutes. The very fact that the conditions required by investigation cannot be simply and rigidly formulated makes it possible and necessary to work creatively under an immense variety of circumstances. From this, research benefits: for it thus gets the advantage of all the suggestions made by practical experience, all the questions propounded by practical difficulties, whether in the class-room, the factory or public life. That any single source of helpfulness or suggestiveness—the university, above all—should be even partially closed may well be deemed preposterous.

That vigorous teaching and unwearying research have flourished together in the German university must in the end be largely ascribed to the elasticity characteristic of the organization. No obstacle obstructs the search of a mature student for a stimulating and congenial teacher; and a teacher with ideas can always gain a hearing for them. It is true that men whose productivity has ceased occupy important chairs in some universities; but in the same institutions, docents with more modern views expound the newer faith, which has perhaps already invaded a professorship somewhere else. While organized faculties tend to relapse into conservatism by favoring their own contemporaries, the pressure of the student body, the legitimate competition of universities with each other on a scientific plane, force the filling of vacant posts with men who represent progressive tendencies. Around such individuals, students of quick susceptibility soon gather; a school forms. The speed with which thereupon a novel standpoint travels over Germany is one of the amazing features of its university life. And this quick apprehension and incorporation of demonstrated truth is responsible for what I have repeatedly pointed out,—the uniformity of the scientific institutes in respect to type, organization, and ideal.

In the field of clinical instruction, Flexner expresses great admiration for the British hospital:

The hospitals and infirmaries in which clinical instruction is given in Great Britain are without exception voluntary institutions, mainly supported by annual subscriptions or gifts and governed by their subscribers through an elective board. The administrative staff is salaried; a few minor medical and surgical posts are modestly remunerated. But the important medical and surgical officers are volunteers, and the insignificant rewards attaching to paid appointments are little more than nominal when viewed in the light of their heavy burden of routine.

It is impossible within the limits of this chapter—and indeed foreign to its purpose—to do full justice to the efforts of these excellent establishments in coping with the formidable problems of disease among the too abundant Scotch and English poor. Suffice it to say that, whether wholly adequate or not, in this cooperative, voluntary endeavor all classes of society loyally and earnestly unite: the nobleman, the merchant, the artisan, together contribute to the funds and assemble to select the managers. No more admirable outlet for civic and social service exists in any modern nation. On the professional side, the spectacle is not less noteworthy: with one or another of the voluntary hospitals all the great names of British medical history have been associated as volunteers; and they are venerated with the intimate pride so charmingly characteristic of British devotion to its past. Harvey was physician to St. Bartholomew's during four and thirty troubled years: the rules governing the kinds of cases admitted to the wards drawn up by him at the request of the governors are followed there to this day. John Hunter, Edward Jenner, and Thomas Young, the last named the expounder of the undulatory theory of light, are among the glories of St. George's: in the board room there, one is still shown the couch on which, prematurely exhausted by his restless labors, Hunter breathed his last. Sir Charles Bell served on the staff of Middlesex; Cheselden was surgeon to St. Thomas's; Sir Astley Cooper to Guy's. On the roll of the Royal Infirmary at Edinburgh can be found the names of all the worthies who built up the medical repute of the university and the extra-mural school,—among others, the Monros, Rutherford, Cullen, James Simpson, and Charles Bell. Nor has this custom ceased to obtain. Our best-known medical and surgical contemporaries have attended or still attend the practice of the voluntary hospitals: Lister at King's, Treves at the London, Horsley at University, Lauder Brunton at St. Bartholomew's, Fraser and Gibson at the Royal Infirmary, Edinburgh.

He goes on to urge that the British medical students' relation to the clinic be adopted universally:

From the preceding account, it is clear that, in the conception of the essentials of clinical discipline, British traditions are thoroughly sound. In all that pertains to the relation of the student to the hospital, the English model deserves to be universally copied.

By the 1930s, most of the American medical schools required an arts degree for admission and had a three- or four-year graded curriculum with clinical instruction and improved hospital facilities. In thirty states, the respective boards of examiners required the prospective doctor to serve a year's internship. As a result of these improvements, the quality of medical education has risen rapidly during the twentieth century.

The dramatic changes in medical education in the United States produced a graduate who changed the face of medical practice. From this point, American medicine could be considered as having joined the mainstream of international medicine.

9

Medicine in the Twentieth Century

TO MARK THE progress of health care—medicine in its broadest sense—chronologically is impossible; many of the roots of modern medicine lie in the nineteenth century, if not earlier.

The shift in emphasis from the health of the individual to that of the group, be it the community or the nation, is seen in a number of advancing fields of medical science. In some instances, community or public health provided early examples of international cooperation that were unrelated to obvious political interests. Jenner's work in developing a vacine for smallpox was the forerunner of international programs of vaccination and inoculation against a variety of agents and the eradication of their intermediate hosts.

Although disease-producing organisms were identified with great rapidity during the latter part of the nineteenth century, their intermediate hosts, or vectors, were not recognized. In 1855, Pettenkofer had postulated that cholera was transmitted by healthy human intermediaries, but the importance of the asymptomatic human carrier was not recognized until almost the close of the century, when a number of investigators indicated that "healthy" carriers were responsible for the spread of such diseases as diphtheria, cholera, meningitis, typhoid, poliomyelitis, and dysentery. The next important step was the identification of nonhuman carriers of parasitic organisms.

Sir Patrick Manson (1844–1922) demonstrated in 1877 that *Filaria bancrofti* was carried by the mosquito, and he postulated such a vector for the malarial parasite. In 1889, ticks were found by Theobald Smith and Kilbourn to be the carriers of the plasmodium of Texas cattle fever, and five years later, David Bruce demonstrated that the trypanosoma, which attacked African cattle, was carried by the tsetse fly. This type of investigation reached a zenith in 1897, when Sir Ronald Ross (1857–1932) discovered that the malarial parasite was carried by mosquitoes (identified by Grassi in 1898 as *Anopheles*). Because malaria at that time was the most prevalent disease, Ross was awarded the Nobel prize for medicine in 1902. Ross went on to direct vigorous campaigns against malaria.

During the nineteenth century, yellow fever often reached epidemic proportions in the southern and eastern parts of the United States almost every summer, and it had foiled the American government's attempts to construct a canal through Central America. Walter Reed (1851–1902), using the observations of Josiah Clark Nott (1804–73) and Carlos Juan Finlay (1833–1915), concluded in 1901 that "the mosquito serves as the intermediate host for the parasite of yellow fever, and it is highly probable that the disease is only propagated through the bite of this insect." The American Medical Corps, led by William Crawford Gorgas (1854–1920), mounted a successful attack on the mosquito, *Aedes aegypti,* in Cuba and Panama. The Rockefeller Foundation Yellow Fever Commission under Gorgas' leadership went on to control the disease in a number of countries in South America.

The discovery of DDT (dichloro-diphenyl-trichloro-ethane) by Swiss scientist Paul H. Müller (1899–1965) was an extremely important advance in the control of insect-borne diseases. Excerpts from his presentation speech when he was awarded the Nobel prize in 1948 summarize the story of his discovery and its importance:

Typhus has always occurred as a result of war or disaster and hence has been named "Typhus bellicus", "War-" or "Hunger-Typhus". During the Thirty Years' War this disease was rampant, and it destroyed the remains of Napoleon's Grand Army on its retreat from Russia. During the First World War, it again claimed numerous victims. At that period more than ten million cases were known in Russia alone, and the death rate was great. Admittedly, the famous Frenchman Nicolle had already, in 1909, shown that the disease was practically solely transmitted by lice—for which discovery he received the Nobel Prize—and thus paved the way for effective control; but really successful methods for destroying lice in large quantities, thus removing them as carriers, were not yet at hand.

Towards the end of the Second World War, typhus suddenly appeared anew. All over the world research workers applied their energies to trying to discover an effective delousing method. Results, however, were not very encouraging. In this situation, so critical for all of us, deliverance came. Unexpectedly, dramatically, practically out of the blue, DDT appeared as a *deus ex machina.*

A research group in Switzerland, under the leadership of Paul Läuger and H. Martin and other collaborators had been engaged since 1933 upon the preparation of oral toxins against textile parasites. This work led to the discovery of a moth-control agent "Mitin" which, on the wool-fibre, looked like a colourless dyestuff. It was discovered at the same time that chemical combinations of the general formula:

Cl ⟨ ⟩ — X — ⟨ ⟩ Cl $X = S, SO, SO_2, O$, etc.

often showed good oral toxicity to moths.

Paul Müller went his own way and tried to find insecticides for plant protection. In so doing he arrived at the conclusion that for this purpose a contact insecticide was best suited.

Systematically he tried hundreds of synthesized organic substances on flies in a type of Peet-Grady chamber. An article by the Englishmen Chattaway and Muir, gave him the idea of testing combinations with the CCl_3 groups, and this then finally led to the realization that dichloro-diphenyl-trichlorome-thylmethane acted as a contact insecticide on Colorado beetles, flies and many other insect species under test. He determined its extraordinary persistence, and simultaneously developed the various methods of application such as solutions, emulsions and dusts. . . .

A number of Swiss research workers such as Domenjoz and Wiesmann now concerned themselves with further trials of the substance. Mooser's researches aimed directly at a prophylaxis of typhus. On the 18th of September 1942, he gave a significant lecture to the physicians of the Swiss First Army Corps, on the possibilities of protection against typhus by means of DDT.

At that time, the Allied Armies of the West were struggling with severe medical problems. A series of diseases transmittable by insects, diseases such as typhus, malaria and sandfly fever claimed a large number of victims and interfered with the conduct of the war. The Swiss, who had recognized the great importance of DDT, secretly shipped a small quantity of the material to the United States; in December of 1942 the American Research Council for Insectology in Orlando (Florida) undertook a large series of trials which fully confirmed the Swiss findings. The war situation demanded speedy action. DDT was manufactured on a vast scale whilst a series of experiments determined methods of application. Particularly energetic was General Fox, Physician-in-Chief to the American forces.

In October of 1943 a heavy outbreak of typhus occurred in Naples and the customary relief measures proved totally inadequate. General Fox thereupon introduced DDT treatment with total exclusion of the old, slow methods of treatment. As a result, 1,300,000 people were treated in January 1944 and in a period of three weeks the typhus epidemic was completely mastered. Thus, for the first time in history a typhus outbreak was brought under control in winter. DDT had passed its ordeal by fire with flying colours. . . .

The application of DDT has also proved effective in the fight against several other diseases transmitted by insects. Thus malaria is spread by several mosquito species. In the fight against malaria, the control of the adult mosquito as well as the larval state form essential part treatments. Under the leadership of Missiroli and the Rockefeller Foundation, large-scale field trials have been held in the old Pontine marshes and in Sardinia as well as in Greece. By simple means excellent results have been obtained there. In consequence the incidence of malaria in these areas has been greatly reduced. In Greece, where before in certain districts 80–85% of the population suffered from malaria, the frequency has been reduced to 5% and the ancient Pontine marshes are now as good as free of malaria.

In DDT therefore, we also possess an extremely valuable remedy in the fight against malaria, this the most widespread of all contagious diseases which yearly affects about 300,000,000 people and causes a yearly death rate of at least 3,000,000. In the cases of many other diseases spread by insects, diseases such as plague, murine typhus and yellow fever, significant results have been obtained.

Just before the end of the nineteenth century, it was recognized that the damage done by a pathogenic micro-organism was not always direct but could result from some toxic substance produced by the organism and carried to other parts of the body. Diphtheria was a dreaded scourge, and investigation into its course was vigorous. In 1889, Yersin and Roux showed that the diphtheria bacillus produced a toxin that circulated in the blood, and Faber found the same thing to be true of tetanus. In 1890, Emil von Behring (1854–1917) discovered that the body developed antitoxins to tetanus, and he actually developed diphtheria antitoxins that could be injected and effectively neutralize the toxins. This discovery not only dramatically reduced mortality from diphtheria but also began a new line of treatment. The production of antitoxins for tetanus and for the venom of various snakes soon followed. Von Behring received the Nobel prize for medicine in 1901. An excerpt from the lecture he gave on that occasion follows:

Since earliest times, in that sphere of medicine which is responsible for the analysis of the symptoms of disease, their cause and natural or artificially induced conquest, namely pathology, humoral and solidistic pathologists have been in opposition to one another. In the last century the solidistic pathologists won the upper hand and the form which Virchow has given to the solidistic pathology by the foundation of *cellular* pathology is now so firmly established that the old humoral pathology can probably be regarded as having been finally laid to rest. With the victory of solidistic *pathology,* however, there has now arrived, pari passu, in the teaching hospitals a solidistic and cellular *therapy* of which one cannot speak so highly as in the case of the cellular *pathology.*

In the treatment of wounds, solidistic trend in therapy expressed itself more in salves, balsams, alteratives, which were supposed to influence the diseased body elements in ill-looking wounds to new and different activity. As you know, this aspect of solidistic therapy has vanished from medicine since Lister, with epoch-making success, laid down the principle, which he taught us to follow down to the smallest detail: "Keep fingers away from wounds, leave the cells as much as possible undisturbed, but take care that noxious agents from *outside* are kept away from wounds and cells".

In internal medicine, however, solidistic therapy remained "faute de mieux". New remedies were constantly coming onto the market and into use in practice which were supposed to curb, with anti-febrins, the vigorous activity of the cells aroused by fever, encourage the will to live and alter the misdirected cell activity. I do not need to quote instances when I maintain that we were all reared in the solidistic- and cellular-therapy dogma according to which the morbid manifestations of life are and must remain the subject of internal therapy. A glance at any Government-sanctioned Pharmacopoeia will show that even now medicaments are classified against a background of this viewpoint.

The detoxicating, or as it is also called, the antitoxic serum therapy, is, on the other hand, *humoral* therapy. Just as little as it has any direct influence on the diphtheria bacilli, is it able to have any direct action, whatever, on the living body elements of the patient who either has, or is threatened with, diphtheria. The detoxicating process acts exclusively in the body *fluids,* in the blood, in the lymphs and in the pericellular lymphatic areas. I must emphasize this especially, because many authors take the view that the diphtheria anti-toxin can also neutralize the poison which has penetrated into the body cells and become established there. My own experience runs entirely contrary to such a view.

Serum therapy in the treatment of diphtheria is, therefore, humoral ther-apy in the strictest sense of the word. It leads us back to the supposedly long-abandoned crasis theory which attributed an important role in the de-velopment and overcoming of disease to the peculiarities of the mixing of the substances solved in the body fluids. As long as there is active diphtheria poison in the body fluids, then a *dyscrasia* exists. After inactivation of the diphtheria poison, or in other words after the detoxication of the body fluids by the addition of diphtheria antitoxin, the *dyscrasia* is overcome; in its place appears, so to say, a *eucrasia*. I do not object if someone tells me that the process of disease does not consist in a faulty mixture of fluids, but in the abnormal functioning of living body elements, the solids of the whole orga-nism. In this sense, there can, in fact, only be solidistic *pathology* or cellular *pathology,* and never humoral pathology since, indeed the lifeless, inert body fluids cannot be attacked by any $\pi\alpha\theta\circ\varsigma$ or illness. In so far, however, as the diseased function of the living body elements is, in the main, conditioned by the incorrect mixture of body fluids, I find the linguistic inconsistency of the use of the word *humoral pathology* no worse than if one speaks of *pathological anatomy,* although the subject matter of this discipline concerns *cadaver* anat-omy and $\pi\alpha\theta\circ\varsigma$ cannot really be attributed to cadavers. However this may be, no one doubts any more of the existence of a humoral *therapy* since antitoxic diphtheria therapy has found an assured place for itself in medicine.

I must add another important epithet to the word *serum therapy* in order to characterize its position in medicine. It is *aetiological therapy* in contrast to the symptomatic therapy just described. As in the case of the Lister treatment of localized wound infections, serum therapy also, in the treatment of general infections, holds to the principle "leave the cells in peace and simply take care that noxious agents from outside are kept out, or, if they once get into the body, are removed".

In the last decade of the nineteenth century, Pasteur discovered preventive inoculation through experiments with the attenuated viruses of anthrax, chicken cholera, and swine measles. The interna-tional traveler today is aware of the availability of inoculations against cholera, yellow fever, typhoid, typhus, and even plague (and, of course, of smallpox vaccination). Under normal circumstances, there is little need for most of these inoculations, but it is unfortunate that the inoculum against tetanus is so often neglected. The most recent addition to these ranks is the poliomyelitis vaccine. Jonas E. Salk (1914–   ), working for the National Foundation for Infantile Paralysis, developed a vaccine against poliomyelitis. In 1952, he inoculated thirty children, who were followed up by Thomas Francis of the University of Michigan School of Public Health. In 1955, Francis declared the vaccination to have been successful. Albert B. Sabin (1906–   ), also supported by the foundation, developed an oral poliomyelitis vaccine by 1959. For some time, the Sabin vaccine was not employed on a large scale, but by 1963, it had for the most part replaced the Salk vaccine. As a consequence of this work, poliomyelitis has been almost eradicated in the United States.

As important as these methods were in attacking the agents of disease, none of them had anything like the significance of chemotherapy. This new field was dominated for several decades by Paul Ehrlich (1854–1915). He was born in the small town of Strehlew in Silesia, where he received his early education, which emphasized Latin and mathematics, at the St. Mary Magdalene Gymnasium. He pursued medical studies at the universities of Breslau, Strasbourg, and Leipzig, receiving a doctorate in medicine at Leipzig in 1878. His doctoral thesis was entitled "Contributions to the Theory and Practice of Histological Colouring," a study that led to modern hematology. During his studies in Strasbourg, Ehrlich successfully used a fuchsin strain to determine if lead were present in tissues. After his appointment to Berlin, he continued to experiment with the relationship between the structure of chemicals and their effects on the body. In 1885, in his study of the oxygen required by organic substances and body tissues, he applied the idea of selective affinity between chemical substances and body tissue to protoplasmic chemistry. From this hypothesis, he arrived at the side chain theory, which postulated that the living protoplasmic molecule consists of a stable nucleus with unstable side chains that enable it to combine with foodstuffs and to neutralize toxins by ejecting detached chains into the blood. This discovery led to immunology. August von Wassermann (1866–1925), whose well-known test for syphilis was first announced in 1906, admitted his dependence on the side chain theory.

During the early part of the century, Ehrlich directed the Royal Institute of Experimental Therapy in Frankfurt. Here he devoted the remainder of his career to problems of immunity and toxins. In 1910, he discovered, in collaboration with his Japanese student Hata, an arsenical compound, Salvarsan, which remained, until the discovery of penicillin, the most widely used drug for the cure of syphilis. Two years previously, he had received the Nobel prize for medicine. The following selection is from a review paper that Ehrlich presented to the Seventeenth International Congress of Medicine in Britain in 1913:

If, e.g., following Castelli, one suspends the spirochaetes of relapsing fever in serum that does not affect their viability, fills two small tubes with the suspension and adds to one of the tubes a very small quantity of salvarsan or neosalvarsan, then centrifuges these suspensions and draws off the liquid, suspends the remaining spirochaetes again in serum and centrifuges once more, then one will obtain in both tubes deposits of spirochaetes which, on microscopic examination, show the same property—equally good motility. If, however, the two deposits of spirochaetes are injected into mice, then one can very soon see that the spirochaetes treated with salvarsan do not give rise to any infection of the animals, while the mice inoculated with the contents of the control tube promptly show signs of infection. This proves that salvarsan, or neosalvarsan as the case may be, is absorbed by the spirochaetes, and must have damaged them, and that this trace of salvarsan, which is so exceedingly minute that it can scarcely be weighed, was sufficient to prevent an increase of the parasites in the animal body. By this very simple and easily intelligible experiment, the direct effect of salvarsan and of anchorage, is proved beyond doubt; the objection that the effect is indirect and based upon antibodies therefore falls to the ground.

It was necessary, however, to go more deeply into the mechanism of this anchorage of medicaments and it is only after long-continued efforts that a clear conception has been obtained. In order to make practical progress it appeared to be necessary not to be satisfied with the basic idea of anchorage as such, but to see in what manner the medicaments are fixed by parasites or by cells. Only by taking a very roundabout way has it become possible to clarify these complicated relationships and in this connexion it was particularly the studies on trypanosomes, above all the investigations of drug-resistant strains, which led to completely unambiguous conceptions of the process of anchorage. There was no difficulty, by continued treatment of the experimental mice with certain compounds, e.g. fuchsin, in finally obtaining a strain of trypanosomes which had become resistant to these compounds, and in the chosen example resistant to fuchsin. There were, in particular, three different classes of compound which were very suited to this purpose:

1. The class of the arsenicals (in the following historical order: arsenious

acid, arsanilic acid (atoxyl), arsenophenylglycine, salvarsan and neosalvar-san).

2. The class of the so-called azo-dyes (the trypan red prepared by Wein-berg, with which Shiga and I experimented, and the trypan blue of Mesnil).

3. Certain basic triphenylmethane dyes (fuchsin, methyl violet, etc.). When a strain of trypanosomes has been rendered resistant to fuchsin, this strain is also resistant to all the substances related to fuchsin and methyl violet, etc., but not to the other classes. Similarly, a strain resistant to arseni-cals is resistant only to arsenicals and not to the two other classes. We see, therefore, that the resistance is of a specific nature, inasmuch as it is limited to a definite class of chemical substances.

This specificity indicated that purely chemical processes are concerned. Earlier studies conducted in a different field, that of the toxins and antitoxins, pointed to the nature of these processes. It was found that the toxins exert their injurious action on the cell by virtue of the fact that they are taken up by certain specific components—side-chains—of the cell, which I have called receptors, and that the antibodies represent nothing more than the cell receptors produced in excess under the influence of the toxin and thrust off.

For many reasons I had hesitated to apply these ideas about receptors to chemical substances in general, and in this connexion it was, in particular, the brilliant investigations by Langley, on the effects of alkaloids, which caused my doubts to disappear and made the existence of chemoceptors seem proba-ble to me.

From this point of view, the phenomena observed in experiments with drug-resistant strains can be readily explained by the fact that the chemocep-tors, under the influence of drug-resistance, suffer an impairment of their affinity, which should be regarded as purely chemical, for certain groups belonging to the drug. This impairment of affinity explains in the simplest possible way why continually increasing quantities of the arsenical become necessary for the destruction, e.g., of a strain of arsenic-resistant trypano-somes, for the reduction in avidity can be overcome only by a corresponding surplus of the arsenical if the quantity necessary for the destruction of the parasites is to be finally anchored.

We therefore come to the conclusion that in the parasites there are present different specific chemoceptors: e.g., and arsenoceptor which anchors the arsenic radicle, an acetoceptor which binds to itself the acetic acid residue, an o-aminophenoloceptor which, e.g., causes the anchorage of salvarsan, and many others. The complete and exhaustive knowledge of all the different chemoceptors of a certain parasite I should like to designate as *the therapeutic physiology of the parasite cell,* and this knowledge is a *sine qua non* for success in chemotherapy. I should like to emphasize that many observations indicate that certain chemoceptors are present in quite different kinds of parasites—

not merely in one alone. The knowledge of these is of especial practical importance, because medicaments which are made to fit them will kill a very large number of widely different pathogenic agents. Therefore, the larger the number of different chemoceptors which can be demonstrated the greater the possibility of successful chemotherapy.

Now, if we are to look for specific medicaments, the first condition is that they must possess a certain definite group which is chemically allied to one of the chemoceptors of the parasites. This is only one of the prerequisites necessary for the medicament to be effective, but generally it is not sufficient in itself. Hundreds of substances may fix themselves to a parasite but only a few are capable of bringing about destruction.

Thus, in the therapeutically suitable substance there must be present, in addition to the anchoring or *haptophore* group, which brings about the fixation, another group which brings about the destruction, and which, therefore, is characterized as the poisoning, or *toxophore* group. This concept exactly corresponds to the views which we have already held for years with respect to the toxins, in which we distinguish the presence of a haptophore group which causes the anchorage to the cell and also the formation of the antitoxins, and a toxophore group which brings about the injurious action on the cell. For the more complicated synthetic medicaments the assumption will have to be made that the haptophore group and the toxophore group are not directly connected with one another, but that they, as residues, are attached, like side-chains, to a chemical molecule. Thus, quite simply, the more complicated chemotherapeutic agents may be compared to a poison-arrow; the anchoring group of the medicament which anchors itself to the chemoceptor of the parasite corresponds to the point of the arrow, the connecting link to the shaft, and the poison group to the arrow poison affixed to the shaft of the arrow. According to this scheme, in salvarsan, dihydroxydiaminoarsenobenzene, the benzene nucleus would correspond to the shaft, the o-aminophenol group to the point, and the trivalent arsenic radicle to the poison.

To continue this comparison, the substances which are used for poisoning the arrows are alkaloids or similar substances which act injuriously on certain vital organs of the body; in the same way we shall have to assume that the toxophore group of the synthetic medicaments poisons the protoplasm of the bacterial cell, and this appears to be possible only if a chemical affinity exists between the toxophore group and constituents of the cell. This view is supported by the fact that all arsenicals containing arsenic in the pentavalent, i.e. fully saturated form, have no therapeutic action, but that this comes about only when the arsenic group is in the unsaturated form, corresponding to the trivalent radicle. The difference between the saturated and unsaturated arsenic radicles has already been brought to light by the veteran-master Bunsen, who, in 1843, in his comparative studies on the non-poisonous cacodylic acid, containing pentavalent arsenic, and the poisonous reduction product cacodyl, containing trivalent arsenic, said that "the cacodylic acid has stopped forming for itself a point of attack by affinity, and thereby, at the same time, has lost its effect on the organism". In the subsequent years a large number of analogous phenomena have, in fact, become known, which speak for the increased activity of unsaturated radicles. The best-known example is doubtless the high toxicity of carbon monoxide as compared with the almost indifferent carbon dioxide. Dyes, only as such, not in the form of their leuco-products which correspond to the saturated state, act as disinfectants. The fact is that all these unsaturated compounds contain unsatisfied avidities which render them capable of additive reaction with other compounds.

In 1908, Ehrlich and Elie Metchnikoff (1845–1916) were jointly awarded the Nobel prize in recognition of their work on immunity. Metchnikoff was born near Kharkoff, Russia, the son of an officer of the Imperial Guard. His interest and ability were so great that he completed the four-year course in natural sciences at the University of Kharkoff in two years. He went abroad for postgraduate study at several institutions, and in 1867, he returned to Russia and held a succession of academic appointments until 1882, when he went to Messina to set up a private laboratory in which he continued his work in comparative embryology and discovered the phenomenon of phagocytosis. Metchnikoff was the first to investigate the question that was central to immunity: How does the body best overcome those pathogenic organisms that have invaded it and established a bridgehead? A summary of his answer to this question is found in the following extracts of his Nobel lecture:

There used to be only a vague answer to the problem of the body's resistance, remarkable as it is. Since the memorable discoveries of Pasteur and his co-workers who found that immunity could be conferred by means of vaccination with microbes, the question has all at once become vastly clarified. The problem has become open to study by experiment. For Pasteur, who was a chemist, the fact that the undamaged organism does not allow certain morbid agents to spread within it, could be explained simply in terms of the chemistry of the environment. In the same way that plants will not grow on soil that lacks some substance indispensable to their growth, so microbes, these microscopic plants which cause infectious disease, are unable to grow in an organism which does not give them all the substances they need.

This theory is completely logical but contradicted a number of factors to be found in the protected organism. Pasteur and his fellow workers realized this themselves when they found that infectious microbes develop very well in the blood of animals that enjoy complete immunity.

The animal organism is very complex and for this reason it is often hard to explain in simple concepts the phenomena to be observed. To achieve the purpose, a different approach has had to be called for. It has been necessary to look from the point of view of biology, and attempt to simplify research conditions without going beyond the scope of the living organism. This is the idea that has been behind our research. Disease is not the prerogative of man and the domestic animals, so it was quite natural to see if the lower animals, with very simple organizations, showed pathological phenomena, and if so, infection, cure and immunity could be observed among them.

To solve medical problems, comparative pathology had to be called in.

While studying the origin of the digestive organs in the animal world, we were struck by the fact that certain of the organism's elements which have no part to play in the digestion of food are nevertheless capable of storing foreign bodies. For us, the reason was that these elements had once been part of the digestive system. This question of pure zoology has no further place here, so we will only stress the general outcome of our research in this field, which was that the elements of the organism of man and the animals, gifted with autonomic movements and capable of enveloping foreign bodies are no more than remains from the digestive system of primitive beings.

Certain of the lower animals, transparent enough to be observed alive, clearly show in their midst a host of small cells with moving extensions. In these animals the smallest lesion brings an accumulation of these elements at the point of damage. In small transparent larvae, it can easily be shown that the moving cells, reunited at the damage point do often close over foreign bodies.

Such observations on the one hand confirmed our assumption on the origin of these migrant elements, while on the other they suggested that accumulation round lesions is a sort of natural defence on the part of the organism. Some method had to be found by which this hypothesis could be verified. I was at this time—more than twenty five years ago—in Messina, so I turned to the floating larvae of starfish, which had been found for the first time on Scandinavian shores and called Bipinnaria. Large enough for several operations, they are transparent and can be observed alive under the microscope.

Sharp splinters were introduced into the bodies of these Bipinnaria and the next day I could see a mass of moving cells surrounding the foreign bodies to form a thick cushion layer. The analogy between this phenomenon and what happens when a man has a splinter that causes inflammation and suppuration is extraordinary. The only thing is that in the larva of the starfish, the accumulation of mobile cells round the foreign body is done without any help from the blood vessels or the nervous system, for the simple reason that these animals do not have either the one or the other. It is thus thanks to a sort of spontaneous action that the cells group round the splinter.

The experiment I have just outlined shows the first stage of inflammation in the animal world. Now inflammation as understood in man and the higher animals is a phenomenon that almost always results from the intervention of some pathogenic microbe. So it is held that the afflux of mobile cells towards points of lesion shows the organism's reaction against foreign bodies in general and against infectious microbes in particular. On this hypothesis, disease would be a fight between the morbid agent, the microbe from outside, and the mobile cells of the organism itself. Cure would come from the victory of the cells and immunity would be the sign of their acting sufficiently to prevent the microbial onslaught. . . .

It has been established as a general rule that in all cases of immunity, natural or acquired, either by preventive vaccination or following an attack of infectious illness, phagocytosis takes place to a marked degree, whereas in fatal or very dangerous diseases, this phenomenon does not exist at all or is attenuated. This rule was demonstrated for the first time on animals immunized against anthrax. When the anthrax bacillus is injected under the skin of sensitive animals, such as the rabbit or the guinea-pig, the microbe is found free in abundant fluid from which the white corpuscles are almost wholly absent. When however the same inoculation is carried out on a rabbit or a guinea-pig that has been previously vaccinated against anthrax, a very different picture results. The bacilli are within a short space of time seized by the white corpuscles which accumulate in quantity at the inoculation point. Once inside the phagocytes, the bacilli die within a comparatively short time. It happens on occasion that only a few hours after the absorption of the bacilli by the white corpuscles, the bacilli are dead.

In time the same rule has been extended to cover a whole host of other infectious diseases. Every time the organism enjoys immunity, the infectious agent falls prey to the phagocytes that gather round the microbes. This general law has even been verified by studying pathogenic microbes, discovered since the law was formulated. With plague, in all cases where the organism is refractory, the plague bacillus is devoured and destroyed by the phagocytes, while in fatal cases of plague the majority of the microbes remain free in the organism's fluids and multiply without hindrance. . . .

The sum of the very numerous facts established in the archives of science leaves no room to doubt the major part played by the phagocytic system, as the organism's main defence against the danger from infectious agents of all kinds, as well as their poisons. Where natural immunity is concerned, and man enjoys this in respect of a large number of diseases, it is a question of the phagocytes being strong enough to absorb and make the infectious microbes harmless. It goes without saying that the phagocytic reaction is helped by every means at the organism's command.

Thus, when the microbes penetrate, the white corpuscles make use of the dilatation of the blood vessels and the nervous actions that control this, in order to reach the battle field in the shortest possible time. Every influence that can trigger off the phagocytosis is naturally brought to bear.

In immunity achieved as a result of vaccinations or subsequent to an attack of the disease, the organism shows a series of modifications. Much stress has been laid on the growth in humoral properties under these conditions. In fact the blood fluid in these cases contains considerable amounts of amboceptors and bacteriotropins (very probably identical) which prepare the microbes for phagocytosis. But, as said above, the amboceptors are products of the phagocytes. Now to secrete great quantities in the humours, the phagocytes must be modified in the organism that has acquired immunity. This might have been expected a priori but it has not been easy to prove by conclusive evidence. Pettersson had the idea of introducing white corpuscles into the organism, originating from animals that had been vaccinated against certain microbes. He found that these elements do give real protection against doses of infectious microbes that are fatal several times over. On the other hand, the white corpuscles of an organism which does not have immunity are powerless to produce this result.

Salimbeni, in view of the outstanding import of this, began a series of experiments at the Pasteur Institute, with the aim of checking Pettersson's findings. Using a method that allowed of great accuracy, he was able to confirm these findings and take them further. He showed that the white corpuscles of the immunized organism are a true source of protective substances, and that at a time when the blood fluid does not yet show any modification. In spite of successive washings, the phagocytes still ensured immunity. In the course of his research, Salimbeni proved that at the moment when the humours have already lost their protective powers altogether, the organism is still refractory and resists fatal doses of infectious microbes. This fact, together with other supporting evidence, leads to a conclusion of the greatest importance. Namely, that even in acquired immunity, the properties of the cells take pride of place over the humoral properties.

Five years later, French physician and physiologist Charles Richet (1850–1935) was similarly honored for his discovery of the reverse of the coin, whose obverse was immunity. He found that in response to exposure to a variety of protein toxins of animal or vegetable origin, at a second exposure of the same degree there was a display of severe toxicity that could be rapidly fatal. When the animal survived, recovery was complete and rapid. This hypersensitivity, which was as constant and as regular as the diminished susceptibility induced by immunization, Richet called *anaphylaxis,* signifying the opposite of *prophylaxis,* or protection.

During the same period, there was considerable interest in another aspect of sensitivity, that is, the agglutinating properties of blood. Karl Landsteiner (1868–1943) was the son of a well-known Viennese journalist and publisher who died when Karl was six years old. He graduated in medicine from the University of Vienna in 1891 and displayed an early interest in immunity and the nature of antibodies. Landsteiner coupled his considerable intellect with the exercise of the greatest care in his scientific observations and descriptions, and this is reflected in his many contributions to morbid anatomy, histology, and immunology. In 1901, he published his discovery that human blood types could be classified into groups according to their different agglutinating properties, and over the next two years, he suggested that this phenomenon of agglutination might be the cause of the shock, jaundice, and hemoglobinuria that had followed some earlier attempts at blood transfusions. He also suggested the value of blood groups in establishing paternity. He received little attention, however, until he classified human blood into the A, B, AB, and O groups in 1901 and pointed out their compatibilities and incompatibilities. Here he tells us of some of his early work:

Owing to the difficulty of dealing with substances of high molecular weight we are still a long way from having determined the chemical characteristics and the constitution of proteins, which are regarded as the principal constituents of living organisms. Thus it was not the usual chemical methods but the use of serological reagents which led to an important general result in protein chemistry, namely to the knowledge that the proteins in individual animal and plant species differ and are characteristic of each species. The diversity is increased still further by the fact that the different organs contain special proteins, and it therefore appears that in living organisms specific building materials are necessary for each particular form and function, whereas man-made machines, performing a wide variety of operations, can be produced from a limited number of substances.

The problem raised by the discovery of biochemical specificity peculiar to a species—the subject of the investigations which we are about to discuss—was to establish whether the differentiation extends beyond the species and whether the individuals within a species show similar though smaller differences. Since no observations whatever had been made in this direction, I selected the simplest experimental arrangements available and the material which offered the best prospects. Accordingly, my experiment consisted of causing the blood serum and erythrocytes of different human subjects to react with one another.

The result was only to some extent as expected. With many samples there was no perceptible alteration, in other words the result was exactly the same as if the blood cells had been mixed with their own serum, but frequently a phenomenon known as agglutination—in which the serum causes the cells of the alien individual to group into clusters—occurred.

The surprising thing was that agglutination, when it occurred at all, was just as pronounced as the already familiar reactions which take place during the interaction between serum and cells of different animal species, whereas in the other cases there seemed to be no difference between the bloods of different persons. First of all, therefore, it was necessary to consider whether the physiological differences discovered between individuals were in fact those which were being sought and whether the phenomena, although observed in the case of blood of healthy persons, might not be due to endured illnesses. It soon became clear, however, that the reactions follow a pattern, which is valid for the blood of all humans, and that the peculiarities discovered are just as characteristic of the individual as are the serological features peculiar to an animal species. Basically, in fact, there are four different types of human blood, the so-called blood groups. The number of the groups follows from the fact that the erythrocytes evidently contain substances (isoagglutinogens) with two different structures, of which both may be absent, or one or both present, in the erythrocytes of a person. This alone would still not explain the reactions; the active substances of the sera, the isoagglutinins, must also be present in a specific distribution. This is actually the case, since every serum contains those agglutinins which react with the agglutinogens not present in the cells—a remarkable phenomenon, the cause of which is not yet known for certain. This results in certain relationships between the blood groups, which make them very easy to determine and which are shown in the following scheme. The groups are named according to the agglutinogens contained in the cells (the sign + in the table indicates agglutination).

Landsteiner continued to investigate blood groups and the chemistry of antigens, antibodies, and other immunological factors found in blood. He must be credited with introducing chemistry into serology. A wide range of immunological investigations have been undertaken since these early discoveries, and research into immunology continues to be very active. Of particular significance is the work of Burnet and

Serum of group	Agglutinins in serum	Erythrocytes of group			
		O	A	B	AB
O	$\alpha\beta$	−	+	+	+
A	β	−	−	+	+
B	α	−	+	−	+
AB	−	−	−	−	−

Medawar. The reaction to tissue grafting stimulated Burnet in 1949 to develop a general theory on the nature of immunity. He felt that there must be a mechanism to distinguish between "self" and foreign material. Although the individual immunological pattern is genetically determined, the ability to produce immunity develops slowly; it is completely lacking in the fetus and is not fully developed until a month or two after birth. Burnet predicted the possibility of experimentally preparing an individual by early exposure to foreign material so as to make him later accept a particular foreign substance as part of self. Medawar and his co-workers were able to prove experimentally the validity of this prediction. This is known as acquired immunological tolerance. Burnet has said, "I like to think that when Medawar and his colleagues showed that immunological tolerance could be produced experimentally the new immunology was born." However, the work of Burnet and Medawar also is of significance in the fields of cancer research and genetics. As with many other biological fields, continuing investigation moves closer to the interface with chemistry as is seen in the work of Edelman in the United States and Porter in the United Kingdom.

The earlier work of Paul Ehrlich in chemotherapy was continued during the 1930s and 1940s both in Germany and in England. Gerhard Domagk (1895–1964), a native of Logan in Brandenberg, received the Nobel prize for physiology and medicine in 1939 for his work on sulfa drugs. Domagk was educated at the University of Kiel, where he received a medical degree in 1921. After a few years as instructor at the University of Münster, he was employed as a researcher by the I. G. Farben Company in Wuppertal. For some years, experiments with gold salts as agents effective against streptococcal infections had been carried out by the Farben Company. At Domagk's suggestion, sulphonamide compounds were among the preparations to be tested. Professor Svartz of the Royal Caroline Institute describes what happened:

During the investigations conducted by Domagk and his co-workers 4-sulphonamide-2', 4'-diaminoazobenzene hydrochloride, among other substances, was tested. This preparation was subsequently named *Prontosil*. The earliest published experiments with Prontosil were begun in December 1932. The lethal dose, for mice, of a certain strain of haemolytic streptococci, which had been isolated from a patient suffering from blood poisoning, had previously been determined. A number of mice were injected with 10 times the lethal dose of this bacterial strain, and approximately half of them were given a specific quantity of Prontosil 1 1/2 hours after being infected.

On 24th December, 1932, it was found that in an experiment begun on 20th December, 1932, all the controls had died, whereas all the mice which had been given Prontosil were alive and well. This was the basis of the discovery which was destined to bring undreamed-of advances in chemotherapy.

The results of these and subsequent experiments, which aroused extraordinary interest, were not published until February 1935, whereupon Prontosil and its effects rapidly became known throughout the world. France was the first country apart from Germany where Prontosil was subjected to practical tests (Levaditi). Extensive experiments on, among other things, the mode of action of Prontosil were then conducted in France (Tréfouël, Nitti), America (Long, Marshall, and others) and Britain (Colebrook, Kenny, and others). One result of these investigations was the discovery that the favourable action of Prontosil was mainly due to the sulphonamide component of the preparation.

Domagk was awarded the Nobel prize in 1939 for his discovery of the antibacterial effects of Prontosil. In 1947, he was cited for further progress in the chemotherapy of bacterial infections. In the following excerpt, he describes this progress:

Within the time at my disposal I can draw attention only to the principal phases in the development of chemotherapy as I see them at present and as they emerge from our work. Even the numerous compounds tested with experimental streptococcal infections during the first phase of the development revealed important laws, which have proved of value to all subsequent workers in the sulphonamide field. It was found, in fact, that only those compounds which contained the sulphonamide group in the *para*-position in relation to the group containing nitrogen were of therapeutic value, whereas compounds with the sulphonamide group in the *ortho-* or *meta*-position were found to be inactive.

Prompted by the German publications on Prontosil—but independently of our own as yet unpublished experiments which were conducted with a view to discovering colourless active sulphonamides outside the azo series-Tréfouël, Nitti and Bovet began to study the same problem. We are indebted to these authors for having drawn attention for the first time in literature to the fact that 4-aminobenzenesulphonamide, which Mietzsch and Klarer had used as initial material for the synthesis of their sulphonamide-containing azo compounds, was therapeutically active as such. This substance was later used in practice as *Prontosil album, Prontalbin,* and *Sulphanilamide.*

It was again Klarer and Mietzsch who initiated a further phase in the development of chemotherapy of bacterial infections by placing at my disposal substances in which the sulphonamide group is no longer unsubstituted, as in the Prontosil compounds, but is modified by an organic radical with replacement of a hydrogen atom. In the case of substances of this type I discovered the action against staphylococci and pneumococci; although there had been a hint of this in Prontosil, which had been reported by me as far back as 1935, it was now considerably increased. Furthermore, I now established for the first time that such compounds, known under the name [Uliron] had a noteworthy effect upon gonococci. The Uliron compounds were the first sulphonamide compounds used in Germany against gonorrhoea after the experiments with Prontosil compounds had proved unsatisfactory.

A further improvement in the action against staphylococci, pneumococci, and gonococci was brought about by introducing a heterocyclic ring in place of the hydrogen in the SO_2NH_2 group. A series of such compounds had already been made available at an early date by Mietzsch and Klarer: however, an intensive study of this field—this time in all advanced countries throughout the world—began only when [Sulphapyridine (p-aminobenzenesulphonamidopyridine)] which had been synthesized by Philipps and Evans, was shown in England by Whitby's experiments to have an effect on pneumococcal infections going beyond that produced by the Prontosil compounds; the broad experience of British clinicians very soon confirmed this experimental finding. This sulphapyridine compound is still in use today in the treatment of lobar forms of pneumonia, but has been superseded more and more by sulphathiazole—subsequently also known by the names Cibazol and Eleudron—which are approximately equally effective against pneumococci and meningococci and still more effective against staphylococci and gonococci, since it very frequently, especially when administered in large doses, causes serious stomach disorders and vomiting. Sulphathiazole or p-aminobenzenesulphonamidothiazole, was produced and a patent was applied for in respect of it independently by several people, but first by Hartmann and Merz. So far sulphathiazole has firmly held its position, although its efficacy in the case of gonorrhoea has progressively declined. For a time people used to speak of a "lightning cure" for gonorrhoea, but ultimately the results became less and less satisfactory although the doses were continually increased. This fact is too well known to require any detailed explanation by me. But we should learn from this undeniable fact and should try to discover the reasons for it. At first the failures were attributed to anatomical causes. People used to speak of the role of sites difficult to reach "Hohlraumeffekt", etc. But this explanation was unsatisfactory and was not sufficient for all cases. Then it was thought that the war might have reduced the patients' resistance, but this explanation likewise did not always hold good. I have constantly emphasized that cooperation by the body is an important factor with any sulphonamide treatment. We all remember how at the beginning of the sulphonamide era it was repeatedly observed that fresh cases of gonorrhoea in men responded best to sulphonamide treatment when suppuration had already occurred for several days, and not at the first appearance of the disease. Perhaps the lowering of natural resistance due to war-time conditions explains why a considerable falling-off in the successes in Germany should to some extent have occurred at a time when optimum results were still being obtained in Switzerland. With the present catastrophic shortage of protein in the diet many patients probably find it difficult to make up the protein losses due to the destruction of leucocytes resulting from an inflammatory condition. However, these facts alone are not sufficient to explain the number of failures. Introduction of resistant strains due to the general upheaval during and after the war was therefore suspected. Finally the question whether gonococci might, like protozoa, possibly become resistant to the drug during treatment was discussed. We ourselves never succeeded in rendering a strain sulphonamide-resistant by treating with small doses of sulphonamide under experimental conditions. However, if this phenomenon should occur in very exceptional cases this would in no way explain the great number of failures. Of decisive importance for a clarification of this question, however, is the fact, which was established by Felke at the beginning of the sulphonamide era, that gonococcal strains of widely differing sensitivity existed from the outset. . . . There can therefore be no doubt that even before the sulphonamide era there were gonococcal strains with a high primary resistance. The resistant strains therefore existed before the sulphonamide era and have not come about as a result of sulphonamide treatment with insufficient doses, or any similar cause. They are due to natural selection. The spread of these resistant strains would have been avoided if the few patients who were carriers of them in 1937 had received careful treatment and had been subjected to clinical supervision until their cure was absolutely certain. But this was not done.

Today we are faced with the same question with regard to the use of penicillin. If we are not to suffer the same disappointment at some future time, the patients with resistant strains must be kept under treatment until they have been definitely cured.

While German scientists opened new fields of chemotherapy, their British counterparts made even more startling discoveries, the most important of which was that of penicillin by Sir Alexander Fleming (1881–1955). Born in Ayrshire, Scotland, Fleming was educated at St. Mary's Medical School in London, where he did research under the guidance of Sir Almroth Wright, a pioneer in vaccine therapy. During World War I, Fleming served as a captain in the Army Medical Corps. He returned to St. Mary's in 1918 and was elected to a professorship in 1928. For his discovery of penicillin, he was elected a Fellow of the Royal Society in 1943. Here, in his own words, he describes his epoch-making discovery:

In my first publication I might have claimed that I had come to the conclusion, as a result of serious study of the literature and deep thought, that valuable antibacterial substances were made by moulds and that I set out to investigate the problem. That would have been untrue and I preferred to tell the truth that penicillin started as a chance observation. My only merit is that I did not neglect the observation and that I pursued the subject as a bacteriologist. My publication in 1929 was the starting-point of the work of others who developed penicillin especially in the chemical field.

Penicillin was not the first antibiotic I happened to discover. In 1922, I described lysozyme—a powerful antibacterial ferment which had a most extraordinary lytic effect on some bacteria. A thick milky suspension of bacteria could be completely cleared in a few seconds by a fraction of a drop of human tears or egg white. Or if lysozyme-containing material was incorporated in agar filling a ditch cut in an agar plate, and then different microbes were streaked across the plate up to the ditch, it was seen that the growth of some of them would cease at a considerable distance from the gutter.

But unfortunately the microbes which were most strongly acted on by lysozyme were those which do not infect man. My work on lysozyme was continued and later the chemical nature and mode of action was worked out by my collaborators in this Nobel Award—Sir Howard Florey and Dr. Chain. Although lysozyme has not appeared prominently in practical therapeutics it was of great use to me as much the same technique which I had developed for lysozyme was applicable when penicillin appeared in 1928.

The origin of penicillin was the contamination of a culture plate of staphylococci by a mould. It was noticed that for some distance around the mould colony the staphylococcal colonies had become translucent and evidently lysis was going on. This was an extraordinary appearance and seemed to demand investigation, so the mould was isolated in pure culture and some of its properties were determined.

The mould was found to belong to the genus Penicillium and it was eventually identified as *Penicillium notatum,* a member of the *P. chrysogenum* group, which had originally been isolated by Westling from decaying hyssop.

Having got the mould in pure culture I planted it on another culture plate and after it had grown at room temperature for 4 or 5 days I streaked different microbes radially across the plate. Some of them grew right up to the mould—others were inhibited for a distance of several centimetres. This showed that the mould produced an antibacterial substance which affected some microbes and not others.

In the same way I tested certain other types of mould but they did not produce this antibacterial substance, which showed that the mould I had isolated was a very exceptional one.

Then the mould was grown on fluid medium to see whether the antiseptic substance occurred in the fluid. After some days the fluid on which the mould had grown was tested in the same way that I have already figured for lysozyme—by placing it in a gutter in a culture plate and then streaking different microbes across the plate. The result is very similar to that observed with lysozyme with one very important difference, namely that the microbes which were most powerfully inhibited were some of those responsible for our most common infections.

This was a most important difference.

By this method and by the method of serial dilution I tested the sensitivity of many of the common microbes which infect us and found that many of the common human pathogens were strongly inhibited while many others were unaffected. . . .

But to return to the properties of penicillin. We had established its specificity. We found that it was of such strength that the culture fluid could be diluted 1,000 times and it would still inhibit the growth of staphylococci. In this connection it is well to remember that phenol loses its inhibitory power when it is diluted more than 300 times. So that in this respect the crude culture fluid on which the mould had grown was three times as potent as phenol.

Then as to its action on the microbe. All the experiments I have cited showed that it was bacteriostatic, that is, it inhibits the growth of microbes. But I showed also that it was bactericidal—that it actually killed them. Then the very first observation of penicillin showed that it induced lytic changes in the bacteria. Thus it was bacteriostatic, bactericidal, and bacteriolytic—properties which have since been shown to be possessed by the purified penicillin. . . .

I had tested all the chemicals which were used as antibacterial agents and they all behaved in the same way—in some concentration they destroyed leucocytes and allowed bacteria to grow. When I tested penicillin in the same way on staphylococcus it was quite a different story. The crude penicillin would completely inhibit the growth of staphylococci in a dilution of up to 1 in 1,000 when tested in human blood but it had no more toxic effect on the leucocytes than the original culture medium in which the mould had been grown. I also injected it into animals and it had apparently no toxicity. It was the first substance I had ever tested which was more antibacterial than it was antileucocytic and it was this especially which convinced me that some day when it could be concentrated and rendered more stable it would be used for the treatment of infections.

Had I been an active clinician I would doubtless have used it more extensively than I did therapeutically. As it was, when I had some active penicillin I had great difficulty in finding a suitable patient for its trial, and owing to its instability there was generally no supply of penicillin if a suitable case turned up. A few tentative trials gave favourable results but nothing miraculous and I was convinced that before it could be used extensively it would have to be concentrated and some of the crude culture fluid removed.

We tried to concentrate penicillin but we discovered as others have done since that penicillin is easily destroyed, and to all intents and purposes we failed. We were bacteriologists—not chemists—and our relatively simple procedures were unavailing, which is not surprising in view of the trouble which the chemists have had with penicillin in recent years.

However, I preserved the culture of the mould and used penicillin habitually for differential culture.

In 1929, I published the results which I have briefly given to you and suggested that it would be useful for the treatment of infections with sensitive microbes. I referred again to penicillin in one or two publications up to 1936 but few people paid any attention. It was only when some 10 years later after the introduction of *sulphonamide* had completely changed the medical mind in regard to chemotherapy of bacterial infections, and after Dubos had shown that a powerful antibacterial agent, *gramicidin,* was produced by certain bacteria that my co-participators in this Nobel Award, Dr. Chain and Sir Howard Florey, took up the investigation. They obtained my strain of *Penicillium notatum* and succeeded in concentrating penicillin with the result that now we have concentrated penicillin which is active beyond the wildest dreams I could possibly have had in those early days.

When these advances in knowledge of microscopic infectious agents and their vectors were occurring, together with the discovery of the means to combat them, other workers were involved in another area that was to be of considerable social consequence. This was in the field of nutrition, where even today there is a great deal to do in public education. We have already seen how Lind's discovery of a cure for scurvy brought about an awareness of the existence of deficiency diseases. Almost a century was to pass, however, before the full impact of this discovery was realized. In 1897, Dutch physician Christiaan Eijkman (1858–1930), working in Java on possible cures for beriberi, found that chickens could be cured of polyneuritis by feeding them either unpolished rice or by treating them with alcoholic extracts of the polishings. It was concluded that beriberi was caused by the lack of some indispensible ingredient in food. Experimentation on human beings led to the same conclusion. In Poland in 1912, little-known biochemist Casimir Funk (1884–1967) discovered that yeast was as effective as rice husks in curing or preventing beriberi. He erroneously concluded that the substance essential for life and growth was an amine and suggested the name "vitamine" to describe it. Meanwhile, Frederick Hopkins in England, Elmer McCallum in the United States, and numerous scientists in continental Europe began a series of experiments that led to the discovery of vitamins ranging from A to T. As a result, such diseases as pellagra, night blindness, scurvy, and rickets are now curable. Rickets, a crippler of children, was discovered to be due to a lack of ergosterol, which could be supplied by vitamin D. The discovery was made in 1927 by German biochemist Adolf Windhaus and the American pediatrician Hess.

Thus far, we have looked at those advances that have been directed toward improved public health. Equally significant scientific advances also were being made with respect to the better diagnosis and treatment of individual patients.

Since the time of Luigi Galvani (1737–98), who showed that electric currents cause muscular contraction, electricity had been used for a variety of ailments, including hysteria, toothache, and deafness. It was the discovery in 1895 of X-rays by German-born Wilhelm Konrad Röntgen (1845–1923) that gave a new role to the use of electricity in medicine and revolutionized methods of diagnosis. As early as 1855, Heinrich Geissler, a scientist at the University of Bonn, had blown tubes that held gases at low pressure and showed a soft glow when a high tension electric discharge was passed through them. Various gases produced different colors. Later in the century, English chemist Sir William Crookes (1832–1919) had shown by deflecting cathode rays by magnet that they were not light, but streams of negative particles possessed of mass.

Röntgen, who was at the time director of the Physical Institute of the University of Würzburg had been using a modified Crookes tube covered with a black cardboard jacket to detect cathode rays. He observed a weak glow shimmering on a nearby bench that moved in unison with the alternating electric discharges he was passing through the tube. Upon closer observation, he discovered that the source of the light was a small fluorescent cardboard screen that he had coated with barium platinocyanide. When he placed his hand in front of the screen, he was able to see the dense shadows of the bone within the outline of the flesh.

Röntgen made his discovery public at the university on January 23, 1896, when he demonstrated that the new rays were not cathode rays but were related to light. He suggested that they be called X-rays in order to distinguish them from other rays and because their real nature was not known. It was not until 1912 that the rays were shown to be of the same character as light, although invisible because of their short wave length. Röntgen, who was given an honorary degree of doctor of medicine by a grateful University of Würzburg in 1896, was also the recipient of the Nobel prize for physics in 1901. Medical use of the new invention was rapid and progressive.

The American physiologist, Walter B. Cannon, while still a student at Harvard, saw the possibilities of using opaque material to study digestive processes in the intestinal tract. In 1895, he delivered a paper entitled "The Movements of the Stomach Studied by Means of the Röntgen Rays," in which he showed how, by the use of bismuth, the stomach could be visualized. Radioactive tracers have been used since the early part of the twentieth century for diagnosis, treatment, and research, but it was not until the middle of the century that radioisotopes were recognized as a valuable tool in diagnosis and prognosis. Other diagnostic inventions of the early twentieth century were the electrocardiograph, devised in 1903 by Willem Einthoven, professor of physiology at the University of Leyden, and the electro-encephalograph invented in 1929 by Hans Berger, director of the psychiatric clinic at the University of Jena. In the same year in Germany, Werner Forssmann (1904–   ) inserted a cannula into his own antecubital vein through which he passed a catheter for 65 cm. and then walked to the X-ray department, where a photograph was taken of the catheter lying in his right atrium. Cardiac catheterization is now a recognized and valuable diagnostic aid.

The first real experiments with the electron microscope were begun in 1928 by Max Knoll and Ernst Ruska of the Berlin Technische Hochschule. They demonstrated that by using a series of magnetic coils electron beams could be used to form a magnified image of the specimen. The first genuine electron microscope, able to surpass optical microscopes in resolution and magnification, was produced by Ruska in 1933.

While these advances greatly improved diagnostic methods, there was parallel progress in the area of therapeutics based on electronics. X rays were used early for the treatment of cancer. The discovery of radium in 1898 by Pierre and Marie Curie opened up a new field: radioactive treatment of cancer. From 1920 to 1930, X rays were used for the treatment of hyperthyroidism. This practice was discontinued when it became apparent that healthy as well as diseased tissue was being destroyed. Radioactive therapy was not used very much after this discovery until after World War II, when radioiodine was substituted for X rays.

Wilhelm Erb (1840–1921), who made the University of Heidelberg a world center for the study of neurology, was the first to use electricity as a diagnostic aid in nerve disorders. Among other contributions in the field of nervous diseases were his descriptions of palsy of the brachial plexus and spastic spinal paralysis. In 1884, Erb gave the first clear description of progressive muscular dystrophy. In France, the clinic of Jean Charcot at Salpetrière attracted students from all over Europe to study nervous disorders. Here hypnosis was successfully applied to the treatment of hysteria.

The development of neurosurgery to complement neurology was another advance at this time, and one of the outstanding figures in the field was Harvey Cushing (1869–1939). He had become interested in neurophysiology as a medical student at Harvard, and after graduation, he assisted Dr. John Elliot (1853–1925) in two operations to remove intracranial tumors. While a surgical resident at Johns Hopkins, Cushing was introduced to a type of neurosurgery characterized by complete control of bleeding and great care and delicacy in the handling of tissue, even though this was only achieved at the sacrifice of speed. After extensive study abroad, he returned to John Hopkins in 1901, where he made brain surgery an acknowledged specialty. Cushing, who became professor of surgery at Harvard in 1911, was the first surgeon to concentrate exclusively on the nervous system, and he carried out extensive research on pituitary function.

Related quite logically to the new interest in neurology was the study and cure of mental disorders. We have already seen how Pinel in the late eighteenth century inaugurated a more liberal approach to the treatment of the insane. This work was furthered in Germany by Wilhelm Griessinger. Born in Stuttgart in 1817, he became director of the famous Charité mental hospital in Berlin in the 1860s. His work, *Pathology and Therapy of Psychic Disorders,* which appeared in 1845, did a great deal to demythologize then-current attitudes toward the insane. It was based upon clinical studies and rational psychological analyses. Griessinger's student Richard von Krafft-Ebing wrote a number of works on psychiatry also based on clinical studies. The most well known of these works was the *Psychopathia Sexualis,* a study of sexual inversion and perversion. Another important aspect of psychiatric study was the work of Ivan Pavlov. Born in Rjazan, Russia, in 1849, he studied in France and Germany. For a time in Leipzig, he was assistant to Carl Ludwig, later the discoverer of the kymograph, who was regarded as one of the leading physiologists of the period. Pavlov's study of the circulation, a field in which Ludwig had specialized, led him to the study of digestion. His early work *Lectures on the Work of the Principal Digestive Glands* won him international recognition. By studying the salivary glands in dogs, he arrived at the notion of the "conditioned reflex."

The physical treatment of mental disease was also advanced by the pioneering work of Julius Wagner von Jauregg (1857–1940), born in Wels in Upper Austria. After receiving his doctorate at the University of Vienna in 1880, he joined the staff of the "Nervein klinik" at his alma mater. Wagner's interest in psychiatry was due in part to the sorry plight of his mother, who suffered from depression most of her life. During the early 1880s, he noticed that certain patients who contracted typhoid fever seemed to recover from their mental afflictions. This observation led to his theory that patients could be cured from psychosis by infecting them with febrile diseases such as malaria or erysipelas. It was not until 1917, when a shell-shocked soldier from the Balkan front arrived at his clinic, that he was able to inoculate others with malarial blood. In June of that year, he injected malarial blood into the bloodstreams of three patients suffering with paresis. The three showed marked improvement soon thereafter, and he published his results. This method of treating general paresis lasted until the introduction of penicillin. Wagner von Jauregg received the Nobel prize for medicine in 1927.

By far the most well known name in the history of early psychiatry is that of Wagner's contemporary, Sigmund Freud (1856–1939). Born in Morania, he moved to Vienna at the age of four. As a student at the University of Vienna, he was at first interested in botany and chemistry. After receiving a degree in medicine in 1881, he worked at the Institute of Cerebral Anatomy, during which time he published a number of articles on neurological pathology. After a period of interest and experimentation with the pharmacologic effects of cocaine in the hope of curing morphine addicts by its substitution, he turned to the study of psychoneurosis. Freud's studies led to the replacement of hypnotism as a means of reviving lost memories by what is termed "free association." The outgrowth is the modern practice of psychoanalysis, or mental catharsis. Three fundamental principles evolved from Freud's studies: the subconscious exists and influences the conscious, the layering of the mind is due to intrapsychical conflict, and infantile sexuality is important. Freud's ideas, especially the interpretation of dreams, soon spread throughout the civilized world and helped to establish psychiatry as the most recent branch of medicine.

Also exciting biologists, and particularly physicians, was the progress made in an understanding of the endocrine glands. As early as the eighteenth century, French physician Théophile de Borden (1722–76) had thought that each human gland produced a secretion that passed into the body and kept the functions of the body in proper balance. Arnold Berthold, a physiologist in Göttingen, Germany, published a study in 1849 that brought the attention of the medical world to the changes that occurred when certain ductless glands were transplanted in chickens. In France, Claude Bernard (1813–78) first used the term "internal secretion" in 1855 in his work on the glycogenetic function of the liver. He wrote that it could be assumed that every tissue, and in general every cell, gives off a certain product that finds its way into the blood and influences all the other cells of the organism. Charles Brown-Séquard (1817–94), who succeeded Bernard as professor of experimental medicine at the Collège de France, provided further knowledge of internal secretions, studying the secretions of the thyroid, adrenals, testes, and pituitary. In 1905, Ernest Starling (1866–1924), who was professor of physiology at University College, London, first coined the term "hormone" to describe internal secretions.

Progress in the new branch of medical science was rapid thereafter. In 1909, it was demonstrated that the parathyroid glands influence calcium metabolism and, three years later, that the posterior lobe of the pituitary gland contained an antidiuretic hormone that controlled diabetes insipidis. The active ingredient of the thyroid was extracted in 1915. It was the isolation of insulin in 1922 by Banting, Best, and Macleod that radically altered the prognosis for diabetes. Here Banting describes the critical experiments:

On October 30th, 1920, I was attracted by an article by Moses Baron, in which he pointed out the similarity between the degenerative changes in the acinus cells of the pancreas following experimental ligation of the duct, and the changes following blockage of the duct with gall-stones. Having read this article, the idea presented itself that by ligating the duct and allowing time for the degeneration of the acinus cells, a means might be provided for obtaining an extract of the islet cells free from the destroying influence of trypsin and other pancreatic enzymes.

On April 14th, 1921, I began working on this idea in the Physiological Laboratory of the University of Toronto. Professor Macleod allotted me Dr. Charles Best as an associate. Our first step was to tie the pancreatic ducts in a number of dogs. At the end of seven weeks these dogs were chloroformed. The pancreas of each dog was removed and all were found to be shrivelled, fibrotic, and about one-third the original size. Histological examination showed that there were no healthy acinus cells. This material was cut into small pieces, ground with sand, and extracted with normal saline. This extract was tested on a dog rendered diabetic by the removal of the pancreas. Following the intravenous injection, the blood sugar of the depancreatized dogs was reduced to a normal or subnormal level, and the urine became sugar-free. There was a marked improvement in the general clinical condition as evidenced by the fact that the animals became stronger and more lively, the broken-down wounds healed more kindly, and the life of the animal was undoubtedly prolonged.

It had been obvious for many years that the ovaries play a greater role in reproduction than the storage and maturation of egg cells.

Allen and Doisy reported during the 1920s that the fluid from ovarian follicles of swine could induce estrous changes in the mouse vagina, but attempts to crystallize the active substance failed. In 1927, Asch-heim and Zondek reported that the urine of pregnant animals contained two hormones, one of which showed activity similar to that of the substance in swine follicular fluid (that is, produced estrus), and the other of which caused significant growth of ovarian follicles. The estrogenic substance in human pregnancy urine, estrone, was crystal-lized in 1929; thus estrogens were the first steroid hormones to be isolated. Androgen crystallization followed two years later.

Studies of the hormones of the adrenal cortex were unsuccessful until the 1930s, when a satisfactory method of adrenalectomy was perfected and when it was recognized that these substances were fat-soluble. Endocrine studies of the pituitary gland were similarly hampered because of the surgical difficulties of removing the pituitary without brain damage. For a long time, it was believed that the pituitary was the "master gland" of the endocrine system. It was the English physiologist Harris, "the father of neuroendocrinology, who not only recognized the subservience of the pituitary to the hypo-thalamus but also established that the neural control of the anterior pituitary was by means of substances secreted into a vascular portal system running between the hypothalamus and the anterior pituitary. Geoffrey Wingfield Harris (1913–1971) was the son of a physicist employed in the Ballistics Department at Woolwich Arsenal who inspired in his son a love of science. He was a distinguished student at Cambridge and St. Mary's Hospital in London, graduating in medicine in 1939. He returned to Cambridge to hold appointments first in anatomy and then in physiology. In 1952, Harris was invited to become the first Fitzmary Professor of Physiology at the University of London, a post that he held for ten years. From 1962 until his death, he was Dr. Lee's Professor of Human Anatomy in the University of Oxford. Here Harris outlines the integrative function of the hypo-thalamus:

In general terms, it is becoming clear that the major role of the hypo-thalamus is to act as an integrative centre. Although the individual pieces of various jig-saw puzzles are doubtless represented at lower levels of the cen-tral nervous system, it is only under the co-ordinating influence of the hypo-thalamus that they are pieced together to give the full pictures of various patterns of behaviour and autonomic adjustment. In many cases these responses are also correlated with particular states of endocrine activity. Thus when, through the control the hypothalamus exerts over the anterior pituitary gland, a female of the lower mammalian species enters the state of oestrus, active copulatory behaviour is linked with the surge in luteinizing hormone which leads to ovulation. In the post-partum female, maternal behaviour, such as nest-building and retrieval and care of the young, is linked with the endocrine changes underlying lactation. The interrelationships of food intake, energy balance and thyroid activity, of fluid intake, control of body-temperature, and the regulation of water excretion (influenced by the posterior pituitary gland) are probably closely linked to produce a stable pattern of metabolism. The important part played by the hypothalamus in co-ordinating autonomic, somatic and endocrine changes necessary for the expression of "sham rage" has long been known.

The evidence that the hypothalamus can act as a "centre" is at the moment incomplete. It is of great interest to know whether a hypothalamic island (consisting perhaps of hypothalamus and septal region), completely separated from all other nervous connexions, is sufficient to maintain oestrous cycles, ovulation and other pituitary-dependent functions. If this is so, then the basic autonomic and endocrine regulation of the hypothalamus would be intrinsic in the structure itself, although open to modulation by other central nervous areas. The diffuse neuronal make-up, and the complex mesh of very fine unmyelinated fibres that constitute a great part of it, probably await the development of new techniques for their analysis. The histochemical analysis of hypothalamic fibre tracts, and the unit recording method applied to hypothalamic neurones, may well be examples of such techniques. . . .

Perhaps related to these preliminary observations is the fact that implants of oestrogenic steroids, which have in themselves a very localized field of action, may result in the same behavioural change when implanted anywhere within a wide area of the hypothalamus. In the same context, the feedback action of gonadal and other target gland hormones on to the hypothalamus poses similar problems of localization and modes of action. The inductive action of testicular hormones in the foetus or neonate, and the excitatory or inhibitory action of these and other hormones in the adult, are open to exploratory studies with radioactive labelled hormones.

In the realm of pure research, perhaps the most exciting advances have been in the field of molecular biology. Although Gregor Johann Mendel (1822–84), the Austrian botanist who became an abbott in the Augustinian order, published in 1866 his hypothesis of the laws of heredity based on careful and thorough experiments with garden peas, the importance of this work was not recognized until 1900. German biologist August Weismann (1834–1914), who was professor of zoology at Freiburg from 1866 until 1912, had maintained that the stability of genetic inheritance through many generations, in spite of innumerable cell divisions, had to have a molecular basis in the living cell. However, it was not until the middle of the twentieth century that the trend toward interdisciplinary investigation, displayed increasingly through the previous fifty years, bore fruit. Here Professor Caspersson of the Royal Caroline Institute outlines the work of the Americans Beadle and Tatum:

The characters, which are transmitted by the genes from generation to generation, present a picture of bewildering multiplicity. This very multiplicity of the genes' effects made it difficult to attack experimentally the problem of their structure and manner of functioning; it was impossible to trace straightforward lines that could serve as a background for an experimental study.

The situation was radically changed by Beadle and Tatum, who, through a daring and astute selection of experimental material, created a possibility for a chemical attack upon the field. Circumstantial evidence pointed to a similarity of the genetic mechanisms throughout the entire plant and animal kingdoms. Beadle and Tatum selected as object for their investigations an organism with very simple structure, a bread mold, *Neurospora crassa,* which is far easier to work with, in many respects, than the objects usually studied in genetics. It is able to synthesize its body substances from a very simple culture medium: sugar, salts, and a growth factor. When cultures of the mold are exposed to X-ray irradiation, mutations—that is, changes in individual genes—result as they do in other organisms. By producing a large number of such mutations and by means of an analysis of the material, which should serve as a model for analytic research, Beadle and Tatum succeeded in demonstrating that the body substances are synthesized in the individual cell step by step in long chains of chemical reactions, and that genes control these processes by individually regulating definite steps in the synthesis chain. This regulation takes place through formation by the gene of special enzymes. If a gene is damaged, for example through irradiation-induced mutation, the chain is broken, the cell becomes defective and may possibly be unable to survive. Even in the formation of comparatively simple substances the steps in the synthetic chain are many, and consequently the number of collaborating genes large. This explains simply why gene function appeared to be so impossibly complex. The discovery provides our best means of penetrating into the manner in which the genes work and has now become one of the foundations of modern genetics. Its importance extends over other fields as well, however.

Especially valuable is the possibility it affords for detailed study of the processes of chemical synthesis in the living organism. In *Neurospora* material it is easy by means of X-ray irradiation to produce quickly a large number of strains in which the function of different individual genes has been disturbed. By comparing these strains we are able to determine in detail how the different stages of synthesis succeed one another when the cell's substances are formed. Beadle and Tatum's technique has become one of our most important tools for the study of cell metabolism and has already yielded results of significance to various problems in the fields of medicine and general biology.

Of equal importance was the X-ray crystallographic characterization of deoxyribonucleic acid by Maurice Hugh Fredrick Wilkins (1916–   ), which led to the "double helix" model of DNA structure proposed by James Dewey Watson (1928–   ) and Francis Harry Compton Crick (1916–   ) in 1953. Since that time, the nature of genetic material and its mode of action have been studied intensively. The significance of Wilkins, Watson, and Crick's work was recognized in the award of the Nobel prize in 1962. The field of cytogenetics is a very active one, and the possibilities of genetic engineering are both fascinating and frightening. Here Crick draws attention to the ubiquity of the twenty amino acids and four bases utilized in the genetic code:

It now seems certain that the amino acid sequence of any protein is determined by the sequence of bases in some region of a particular nucleic acid molecule. Twenty different kinds of amino acid are commonly found in protein, and four main kinds of base occur in nucleic acid. The genetic code describes the way in which a sequence of twenty or more things is determined by a sequence of four things of a different type.

It is hardly necessary to stress the biological importance of the problem. It seems likely that most if not all the genetic information in any organism is carried by nucleic acid—usually by DNA, although certain small viruses use RNA as their genetic material. It is probable that much of this information is used to determine the amino acid sequence of the proteins of that organism. (Whether the genetic information has any other major function we do not yet know.) This idea is expressed by the classic slogan of Beadle: "one gene—one enzyme", or in the more sophisticated but cumbersome terminology of today: "one cistron—one polypeptide chain".

It is one of the more striking generalizations of biochemistry—which surprisingly is hardly ever mentioned in the biochemical textbooks—that the twenty amino acids and the four bases, are, with minor reservations, the same throughout Nature. As far as I am aware the presently accepted set of twenty amino acids was first drawn up by Watson and myself in the summer of 1953 in response to a letter of Gamow's.

Cancer is a major interest of scientists of diverse backgrounds, and the wide range of disciplines involved in cancer research has greatly increased our knowledge of this scourge. In the early 1960s, Francis Peyton Rous, working in the United States, discovered viruses capable of producing tumors, and Renato Dulbecco, working in the United Kingdom, developed laboratory techniques that enabled research workers to study the molecular biology of animal viruses with great precision. Ten years later, two Americans, David Baltimore and Howard M. Temin, discovered a unique enzyme that reverses the flow of genetic information that would normally run from DNA to the messenger RNA, thus providing a mechanism for viruses to establish themselves as parts of normal cells and change the cell's growth rate.

The twentieth-century movement toward the interfaces between traditional scientific disciplines has not only allowed biological sciences to make use of physics, biochemistry, and computer analysis, for example, but also has led to a changed philosophy of man's place in the scheme of things. This is demonstrated graphically by a comparison between the attitudes of two great medical thinkers and distinguished scientists: Thomas Henry Huxley (1825–95) and Sir Charles Scott Sherrington (1861–1952). Huxley's view of the central question in biological enquiry during the nineteenth century can be summed up in the title of one of his papers published in 1863 *Man's Place in Nature*, whereas Sherrington pointed up the changed emphasis of twentieth-century endeavors by turning the phrase, "Man on his nature."

Perhaps this change in philosophy, carrying with it, as it does, the realization that man is a part of nature and changes with it, rather than being a detached observer, is the single most significant factor in contemporary medical history. The obvious effect of this change has been an increasing social awareness of the problems of population control, aging, and the cost of restoration and maintenance of good health.

The unprecedented increase of births over deaths began during World War II, chiefly as a result of disease control, and the rate of population growth rises more steeply each year. The world population grew slowly over thousands of years until it reached 1 billion in 1825. However, the second billion was added in just over one hundred years (by 1930), and the pace continues to quicken so that the 3 billion mark was reached in 1960, and it is predicted that the world population will reach 4 billion by 1980 or shortly thereafter. Advancing hand in hand with this population growth is ever-increasing urbanization, with the concomitant strain upon housing, water supply, sewage facilities, and other hallmarks of urban life. Thus, man's advances in the control of death have inexorably brought him in conflict with the issue of control of birth.

Birth control, through abortion and by means of physical and chemical contraceptives, has been practiced throughout recorded history, but it is only since steroidal contraceptives became readily available in the twentieth century that family planning became possible on a wide scale. The science of endocrinology did not become established until this century, and much of the work has been with reproductive hormones. From the turn of the century, it had been known that extracts from the corpus luteum prevented ovulation following injection into various animals. By 1935, investigators had identified what was believed to be the active substance of the corpus luteum, its clinical structure was known, it was possible to make it synthetically from readily available steroids, and the world had agreed on a name for it: progesterone. Synthetic steroids were developed with some of the biological activities of progesterone, and after several independent investigators had developed a group of compounds, known as the 19-norsteroids, which had potent progestational activity, there developed a strong impetus toward the development of a practical oral contraceptive that inhibited ovulation. The first large-scale employment of an oral contraceptive was undertaken by Rock and Pincus at the Family Planning Center in Puerto Rico. This work, and a major study in 1956 by the staff of the Los Angeles Planned Parenthood Center supported by the Population Council, firmly established the effectiveness of oral contraception with steroids.

One of the by-products of the advances made in twentieth-century medicine has been the increasing age of the population. The cure of childhood diseases and the increasing knowledge of cancer and other degenerative diseases have of course been partially responsible for this. But it is largely a result of the economic and social changes of the twentieth century. Whereas at the beginning of the century less than 4 percent of the U.S. population was over sixty-five the proportion today is 10 percent, and by the beginning of the next century, it is estimated that 25 percent will be sixty-five or older. The term "geriatrics," which refers to the diseases of old age, was first used by the American Nascher in 1916, but a concern for the diseases of the aged is found throughout the entire history of medicine. As a result of the discovery of DNA, containing as it were the blueprints that make man what he is, scientists now speculate about the causes of aging. Some regard the aging process as part of a genetic master plan imprinted in the cells, whereby at the end of a certain period of time certain cells no longer reproduce. It has been demonstrated that after about the age of thirty massive numbers of brain cells die daily and a similarly significant atrophy is true of the taste buds. Another theory holds that man ages because the program contained in the DNA molecules becomes erratic with the passage of time. It is generally agreed that the brain has a role to play in the aging process, particularly the hypothalamus. The enzyme monoamine oxidase, which breaks down biogenic amines associated with nerve impulses, has been found to increase in the brain after the age of forty-five. This high level of monoamine oxidase may cause the hypothalamus to signal a slowing down of endocrine activity, resulting in the aging process.

Whatever the nature of the process, we know so little about it that it is not possible to distinguish acceptable limits of normal change, thereby defining what pathological changes are associated with old age. Recently, the United Kingdom has taken the lead in developing a systematic and comprehensive approach to the problems of aging based on the pioneering work of such men as T. H. Howell and the establishment of gerontology research centers, but there is a long way to go.

In New Zealand, government assistance in health care began with the creation of a national hospital system that began with the Colonial Hospitals built by Governor Sir George Grey in various centers of colonial settlement. The first of these, the Auckland Hospital, was begun in 1846 and admitted patients even before the upper story was completed. These hospitals were intended for the native Maori population and for the British settlers; in addition to the admission of Maori patients, many more were treated as outpatients.

The first Hospitals and Charitable Institutions Act was passed in 1885 and set the pattern for a hospital system that in the main has continued up to the present. The country was divided into twenty-eight hospital districts, each controlled by a board whose members were appointed annually by local authorities. The hospitals were to be financed by patient fees, and, it was hoped, by voluntary contributions, the balance being supplied by local rates with a government subsidy. A number of "separate institutions," which also received money from the rates as well as government subsidies, continued independently so that in effect there were two separate systems existing together. A new act was passed in 1909 under which board members were elected to a three-year term by the voters of their district. All the separate institutions that could not operate without assistance from the local ratepayers were taken over by the hospital boards, and the number of hospital districts was increased to thirty-six.

By 1926, when the third major hospitals act was passed, the number of hospital districts had been further increased, and the boards received approximately one-third from local rates and one-third from a government subsidy.

The act of 1926 remained in force for thirty-one years, by which time the method of financing the hospitals had undergone such great changes that the Hospitals Act of 1957 became necessary. The introduction of hospital benefits under the Social Security Act 1938 relieved patients of the payment of fees, while in 1946, the maximum rate of hospital board levy on local authorities was established at one half-penny per pound of the rateable capital valuation. From 1951 to 1957, this was still gradually reduced until hospital income from local rates was entirely abolished and the government became responsible for all public hospital finance.

Sweden established its System of Medical Care and Sickness Benefit Insurance, on January 1, 1955. Compulsory participation is required of all citizens, and costs are divided among employer, employee, and government. Doctors are not employed by the government, but the government regulates physician and hospital fees.

Saskatchewan, Canada, began its Medical Care Insurance and Hospital Services Plan in 1962. This enables residents to obtain insurance covering many medical services. This government-administered program is funded by an annual tax and by the use of federal funds from the Canadian government.

In the United States, a limited form of health insurance, Medicare, is available to the elderly and to certain disabled persons. This federal program has two parts: the first provides hospital insurance, which extends to nursing homes and home health agencies, and the second provides medical insurance, assists in paying doctors and certain hospital outpatient services. The individual pays part of the cost of many services provided under Medicare, and in general, these amounts increase as general health care costs rise. Inability to pay these amounts in some cases leads to assistance from state Medicaid programs, which itself is subsidized with federal funds.

The growing conviction, which is almost universal today, that we have a responsibility for our fellow beings is expressed in a variety of ways that are related to health. One is the growth of "socialized medicine," which flourishes worldwide in one form or another. This conviction also is expressed in the concern with our environment and the vigorous efforts to combat pollution.

The development of agencies concerned with funding medical research is characteristic of the twentieth century. Both government agencies and private foundations have made significant contributions to medical progress. However, such agencies direct research by funding particular areas of inquiry at the expense of others. And this is not necessarily in the best public interest. Increasingly, however, society will take an interest in progress in health care, in particular, the growing concern in prevention rather than cure.

Cooperation between nations has been particularly noticeable since World War II, but the foundations for the World Health Organization (WHO) were probably laid over one hundred years ago. In 1839, Sultan Mahmoud II of Turkey, concerned with epidemic diseases, established a quarantine system for the Ottoman Empire that led to an international organization to enforce sanitary regulations. This Conseil Supérieur de Santé de Constantinople had sixty-three health offices and was independent of local Turkish health offices.

The first International Sanitary Conference was held in Paris in July 1851, and these conferences continued into the twentieth century. The eleventh conference, in 1903, succeeded in developing an instrument with provisions related to cholera and plague. It is surprising that no provision was made for yellow fever, particularly because the mode of transmission had been recently discovered. In 1902, the International Sanitary Bureau for the Americas had been established to eradicate yellow fever. The conference of 1903 proposed a new international organization, which led, in 1907, to the foundation of the Office International d'Hygiène Publique with its headquarters in Paris. The office made numerous studies related to communicable diseases and public health and published a monthly bulletin. In 1920, the League of Nations Health Organization was established, and both institutions co-existed until they were absorbed into WHO, which was set up in 1946. WHO also absorbed the temporary organization, United Nations Relief and Rehabilitation Administration, which was instituted immediately after World War II to meet urgent needs.

In June 1948, the first World Health Assembly, headquartered in Geneva, set about preparing a program of work. It was decided that most of its activities would be undertaken on a regional basis. There is a regional committee composed of representatives of governments in the area and a regional office staffed by a WHO secretariat with a director. The World Health Assembly is the only place in which all member states are directly represented. It determines policy and makes recommendations to member states. It instructs the executive board and the director general and is responsible for the finances of the organization. The annual meeting of the assembly is both a business meeting and an opportunity for technical discussions.

The program of the World Health Organization is governed by five basic principles:

1. Participation by all countries.
2. Assistance only upon governmental request.
3. Assistance should be appropriate to the total environment of the people being helped and should foster self-reliance.
4. Research efforts should be restricted to support of current work.
5. Assistance should be available to all member states.

The WHO program changes to reflect the changing needs of its member states, particularly those of developing countries. One of the major areas of activity, public health administration, covers the training of professional, paramedical, and auxiliary workers; the provision of teams to help develop health services; and assistance to existing services such as public health laboratories and rehabilitation centers.

Another area, environmental health, provides planning and development of water supplies and sewage disposal, trains sanitary engineers and other workers, and attacks the many problems that accompany population growth and urbanization. In addition to other endeavors, there is an ongoing program of disease control and eradication.

International organizations are often viewed with suspicion, particularly with regard to the degree of objectivity employed in developing and implementing their programs. The World Health Organization is respected and has an enviable reputation for integrity and competence, and there is so much for WHO to do that its impact on health in the coming years could be very great indeed. Unfortunately, not all countries are prepared to participate, and some that do allow political considerations to influence policy decisions. The extent to which these drawbacks can be overcome will determine the effectiveness of WHO.

The rate that knowledge is being acquired means that a history such as this cannot include all the advances in medical science. It has been necessary to select those things that appear to be of the greatest significance to mankind and to ignore other advances, such as organ transplant or computer application, which are considerable scientific achievements. This same growth of knowledge makes it almost impossible to predict future interests and goals.

In the seventeenth century, scientists such as Galileo, Bacon, Descartes, Newton, and others expected that the development of a new "natural philosophy" based on observation and reasoning would lead to man's control of nature. Unfortunately, this has not been the case. Observation and reasoning have proceeded satisfactorily, with tremendous scientific advances, but this has not resulted in man's control of nature. Indeed, the new knowledge has made the interdependence of man and nature very clear. Moreover, there is a price for the advances, for example, the antibiotics that eradicate disease also have led to the development of resistant strains. New technological advances require accompanying philosophical and ethical advances, for example, the way in which genetic engineering will be handled. It is generally agreed that the development of philosophical and moral concepts to match our scientific advances is the area of greatest need and least progress.

References and Selected Readings

The authors have relied on a wide range of primary and secondary sources. Of significant importance has been the work of Walter Artelt, *Einfuhrung in die Medizinhistorik, ihr Wesen, ihre Arbeitsweise und ihre Hilfsmittel* (Stuttgart, 1949). Max Neuberger's *Geschichte der Medizin*, 2 vols. (Stuttgart, 1906–11), has been utilized for accounts of ancient and medieval medicine as has the more recent work of F. Diepgen, *Geschichte der Medizin*. For modern European medical history, there has been some reliance on the classic work of Arturo Castiglioni, *Storia della medicine*. Even in cases where earlier translations from the medical works of antiquity were available, the modernization was based on the critical editions of the *Corpus Medicorum Graecorum* and the *Corpus Medicorum Latinorum*. Because our selections were of necessity limited, we recommend to the reader interested in a wider selection *Medical Classics*, E.C. Kelly, ed., 5 vols. (Baltimore, 1936–41). We list below references and recommended readings for each chapter.

1 PREHISTORY AND ANCIENT CIVILIZATIONS
D. Bothwell, *Diseases in Antiquity* (Springfield, 1967).
B. Ebbell, *The Papyrus: The Greatest Egyptian Medical Document* (Copenhagen, 1939).
S. Glanville, *The Legacy of Egypt* (Oxford, 1942).
B. Gordon, *Medicine Throughout Antiquity* (Philadelphia, 1949).
E. Hume, *The Chinese Way of Medicine* (Baltimore, 1940).
W. Jaywe, *The Healing Gods of Ancient Civilization* (New Haven, 1925).
H. Sigerist, *A History of Medicine, Vol. I, Primitive and Archaic Medicine* (Oxford, 1951).
R. Thompson, *The Devils and Evil Spirits of Babylonia* (London, 1903).
H. Zimmer, *Hindu Medicine* (Baltimore, 1948).

2 HELLENIC MEDICINE
R. Caton, *Temples and the Ritual of Asklepios at Epidaurus and Athens* (London, 1900).

M. Clageit, *Greek Science in Antiquity* (New York, 1956).
L. Edelstein, *The Hippocratic Oath* (Baltimore, 1943).
S. Elliot, *Outline of Greek and Roman Medicine* (London, 1914).
H. Kitto, *The Greeks* (Baltimore, 1951).
G. Majno, *The Healing Hand* (Cambridge, 1975).
S. Sambursky, *The Physical World of the Greeks* (London, 1956).
C. Singer, *Greek Biology and Medicine* (Oxford, 1922).

3 HELLENISTIC MEDICINE
T. Allbutt, *Greek Medicine in Rome* (London, 1921).
J. Carcapino, *Daily Life in Ancient Rome* (New Haven, 1940).
L. Cohn-Haft, *The Public Physicians of Ancient Greece* (Vol. 42, Smith College Studies in History, 1956).
C. Harris, *The Heart and the Vascular System in Ancient Greek Medicine from Alcmaeon to Galen* (Oxford, 1973).
M. Rostovtzeff, *The Social and Economic History of the Hellenistic World* (Oxford, 1941).
G. Sarton, *Galen of Pergamon* (Lawrence, 1954).
_____*A History of Science: Hellenistic Science and Culture in the Last Three Centuries, B.C.* (Cambridge, 159).
C. Singer, *Greek Biology and Medicine* (Oxford, 1922).
W. Torn, *Hellenistic Civilization* (New York, 1952).

4 THE MIDDLE AGES
F. Bratton, *Maimonides "Medieval Modernist"* (Boston, 1967).
L. Brehier, *La civilization Byzantine* (Paris, 1950).
R. Carton, *Chez Roger Bacon* (Paris, 1924).
_____*L'experience physique* (Paris, 1929).
L. Gauthier, *Ibn Roschd* (Paris, 1948).
A. Goichon, *Ibn Sina* (Paris, 1933).
C. Haskins, *The Renaissance of the Twelfth Century* (Cambridge, 1927).
J. Minkin, *The World of Maimonides* (New York, 1957).
F. Oakley, *The Medieval Experience* (New York, 1974).
D. O'Leary, *Arabic Thought and Its Place in History* (London, 1922).
D. Reismon, *The History of Medicine in the Middle Ages* (New York, 1935).
G. von Strunebaum, *Medieval Islam* (Chicago, 1953).
A. Vasiliev, *History of the Byzantine Empire*, 2 vol. (Madison, 1952).
J. Wohl, *The Black Death* (London, 1926).

5 THE RENAISSANCE
M. Boas, *The Scientific Renaissance, 1450–1630* (London, 1962).
E. Chamberlain, *Everyday Life in Renaissance Times* (New York, 1965).
M. Crosland, *Historical Studies in the Language of Chemistry* (London, 1962).
C. O'Malley, *Andreas Vesalius of Brussels* (Berkeley, 1965).
W. Pagel, *Paracelsus: An Introduction to Philosophical Medicine in the Era of the Renaissance* (New York, 1958).

REFERENCES AND SELECTED READINGS 225

F. Pellegrini, *Fracostoro* (Trieste, 1948).

R. Taton, ed., *The Beginnings of Modern Science from 1450 to 1800* (London, 1964).

G. Whiteridge, *William Harvey and the Circulation of the Blood* (New York, 1971).

W. Wightman, *Science and the Renaissance* (Edinburgh, 1962).

6 THE AGE OF THE ENLIGHTENMENT

E. Cassirer, *The Philosophy of the Enlightenment* (Boston, 1961).

G. Clark, *Science and Social Welfare in the Age of Newton* (New York, 1949).

P. Delaunay, *La view medicale aux 16ème, 17ème, et 18ème siècles* (Paris, 1935).

K. Dewhurst, *Dr. Thomas Sydenham (1624-1689)* (Berkeley, 1966).

R. H. Fox, *William Hunter: Anatomist, Physician, Obstetician (1718-1783)* (London, 1901).

P. Hazzard, *The European Mind* (New York, 1959).

L. King, *The Medical World of the Eighteenth Century* (Chicago, 1958).

J. Kobler, *The Reluctant Surgeon: Biography of John Hunter, Medical Genius and Great Inquirer of Johnson's England* (Garden City, N.Y., 1960).

W. LeFanu, *A Bio-Bibliography of Edward Jenner* (Philadelphia, 1951).

G. Lindeboom, *Herman Boerhaave: The Man and His Work* (London, 1968).

M. Ornstein, *The Role of Scientific Societies in the 17th Century* (New York, 1939).

J. Vrooman, *René Descartes* (New York, 1970).

W. Wartman, *Medical Teaching in Western Civilization* (Chicago, 1970).

7 MEDICINE IN INDUSTRIALIZED SOCIETY

E. Ackerbnecht, *Rudolf Virchow* (Madison, 1953).

T. Bilbroth, *The Medical Sciences in the German Universities* (New York, 1924).

M. Buer, *Health, Wealth, and Population in the Early Days of the Industrial Revolution* (New York, 1968).

W. Bullocch, *The History of Bacteriology* (London, 1938).

R. Dubos, *Louis Pasteur* (Boston, 1950).

D. Guthrie, *Lord Lister* (Baltimore, 1949).

S. Harris, *Woman's Surgeon: The Life of J. M. Sims* (Newark, 1950).

L. Hober, *The Chemical Industry in the 19th Century* (New York, 1958).

E. Hume, *Max von Pettenbofer* (New York, 1927).

R. Lewis, *Edwin Chadwick and the Public Health Movement, 1832-1854* (London, 1952).

G. Miller, *Adoption of Inoculation for Smallpox in England and France* (Philadelphia, 1957).

J. Olmsted, *Claude Bernard* (New York, 1928).

R. Sand, *Vers la medicine sociale* (Paris, 1948).

H. Shryock, *The Development of Modern Medicine* (New York, 1942).

8 MEDICINE IN THE AMERICAS

J. Burrow, *AMA: Voice of American Medicine* (Baltimore, 1963).

K. Dewhurst, *Dr. Thomas Sydenham: His Life and Original Writings* (Berkeley, 1966).

J. Duffy, *Epidemics in Colonial America* (Baton Rouge, 1853).

G. Grob, *The State and the Mentally Ill* (Chapel Hill, N.C., 1966).

F. Marti-Ibanez, ed., *History of American Medicine: A Symposium* (New York, 1959).

A. Moll, *Aesculapius in Latin America* (Philadelphia, 1944).

F. Packard, *History of Medicine in the United States,* 2 vols. (New York, 1963; reprinted from 1931 edition).

C. Rosenberg, *The Cholera Years* (Chicago, 1968).

R. Shryock, *Medicine in America: Historical Essays* (Baltimore, 1966).

H. Sigerist, *American Medicine* (New York, 1934).

J. Young, *The Medical Messiahs: A Social History of Health Quackery in Twentieth-Century America* (Princeton, 1967).

9 MEDICINE IN THE TWENTIETH CENTURY

L. Bickle, *Rise Up to Life: A Biography of Howard Walter Florey, Who Gave Penicillin to the World* (New York, 1972).

J. Butler, *Science and Human Life* (New York, 1957).

E. Curie, *Marie Curie* (New York, 1937).

E. Farber, *Nobel Prize Winners in Chemistry, 1901–1961* (London, 1963).

I. Gladston, *Behind the Sulfa Drugs* (New York, 1943).

O. Glaser, *Dr. W. C. Roentgen* (Springfield, 1945).

P. de Kruif, *The Microbe Hunters* (New York, 1932).

A. Newsholme, *The Story of Preventive Medicine* (Baltimore, 1929).

S. Riedman, *Portraits of Nobel Laureates in Medicine and Physiology* (New York, 1963).

A. Sayre, *Rosalind Franklin and DNA* (New York, 1957).

B. Sokoloff, *The Story of Penicillin* (New York, 1945).

L. Stevenson, *Nobel Prize Winners in Medicine and Physiology, 1901–1950* (New York, 1953).

L. Teleky, *History of Factory and Mine Hygiene* (New York, 1948).

J. Watson, *Double Helix: Being a Personal Account of the Discovery of the Structure of DNA* (New York, 1968).

C. Winslow, *The Conquest of Epidemic Disease* (Princeton, 1943).

Important Dates
in the History of Medicine

1500 B.C.—Ebers papyrus
1300 B.C.—Berlin papyrus
800 B.C.—Brahminic medicine
  practiced
600 B.C.—Chinese practiced
  acupunture and massage
460 B.C.—Birth of Hippocrates
400 B.C.—Description of Athenian
  epidemic by Thucydides
31 B.C.-A.D. 14—Celus, *De Re Medica*
55-63—Lucretius describes epidemic
  in *De Rerum Natura*
848-856—School of Salerno
860-932—Rhazes
980-1037—Avicenna
1135-1204—Moses Maimonides
1139—Lateran Council interdicts
  surgery among the higher clergy
1181—Montpellier declared a free
  school of medicine
1197—St. Mary's Spital in London
1214—Bologna hires Ugo Borgognoni
  as city physician
1218—Collège de St. Come founded
  at Paris by Jean Pitard
1224—Federick II issues law
  regulating the study of medicine
  and founds University of Messina
1231—Salerno constituted a medical
  school by Federick II. Federick II

issues law authorizing a
quinquennial dissection and
pharmacy.
1247—Council of LeMans prohibits
  surgery to monks
1267—Council of Venice forbids Jews
  to practice medicine among
  Christians
1285—Salvino degli Armati invents
  spectacles
1295-96—Lanfranc completes his
  treatise on surgery
1300—Boniface VIII issues bull *De
  Sepulturis*
1315—Mondino makes his first public
  dissection of a human subject
1317—John XXII issues bull *Spondent
  Pariter* against abuses of alchemy
1333—Public medico-botanical garden
  at Venice
1348—Board of Health and quarantine
  established at Venice
1348-50—Black Death
1363—Guy de Chauliac completes his
  Chirurgia magna
1376—Board of medical examiners in
  London
1388—Salaried city veterinarian in city
  of Ulm
1391—University of Lerida permitted

to dissect a body every three years

1404—First public dissection at Vienna

1450—Nicholos of Cusa suggests timing the pulse and weighing blood and urine

1457—Purgation—Calendar printed by Guttenburg (first medical publication)

1493—Birth of Paracelsus

1495—Maximilian I issues Edict against Blasphemers (first mention of syphilis)

1508—Guaiac wood brought from America

1514—Birth of Vesalius

1524—Cortes erects first hospital in city of Mexico

1530—Fracastoro poem on syphilis published

1540—English barbers and surgeons united as "Company of the Barbers Surgeons"

1543—Vesalius publishes the *Fabrica* and founds modern anatomy

1561—Fallopius publishes his *Observationes Anatomicae*

1564—Eustachius discovers nerve and suprarenal glands

1567—Paracelsus' account of miners' phthisis published

1582—University of Edinburgh chartered by James VI

1590—Invention of compound microscope by Johannes and Zacharias Jansen

1603—Prince Cesi founds the Accademia dei Lincei at Rome

1620—Van Helmont teaches that a chemical substance survives in its compounds

1628—Harvey publishers *De Motu Cordis*

1635—Richelieu founds the Academic Française

1636—Harvard College founded by act of General Court of Massachusetts Assembly of Virginia

passes act regulating physicians' fees

1637—Descartes shows that accommodation depends on change in the form of lens

1648—Francesco Redi disproves the theory of spontaneous generation

1657—Accademia del Cimento founded at Florence

1658—Swammerdam describes red blood corpuscles

1659—Malpighi outlines lymphadenoma, or Hodgkin's disease

1660—Malpighi discovers anastomosis between capillaries

1661—Robert Boyle defines chemical elements

1664—Swammerdam discovers valves of lymphatics

1679—Nicholas de Blegny publishes the first medical periodical

1680—Leeuwenhoek discovers yeast plant

1680-81—Borelli's *De Motu Animalium* published

1686—Sydenham describes chorea minor

1700—Ramazzini publishes treatise on trade diseases

1703—Leeuwenhoek discovers parthenogenesis of plant lice

1732—Boerhaave's *Elementa Chemiae* published

1735—Linnaeus' *Systema Naturae* published

1754—Van Swieten organizes clinical instruction in Vienna

1757—Lind's treatise on naval hygiene published

1766—Cavendish discovers hydrogen

1770—William Hunter founds school of anatomy in Great Windmill Street

1771—Priestly and Scheele isolate oxygen

1772—Rutherford discovers nitrogen

Priestly discovers nitrous oxide
1774—Scheele discovers chlorine
1775—Lavoisier discovers and defines oxygen
1777—Lavoisier describes exchange of gases in respiration
1778—John Hunter's treatise on diseases of the teeth published
1780—Rush describes dengue
1786—John Hunter publishes *Treatise on the Venereal Disease*
1789—Medical Society of South Carolina founded
1792—Galvani's essay on animal electricity published
1798—Jenner's *Inquiry* published
1800—Davy discovers anesthetic effect of laughing gas
1801—Pinel publishes psychiatric treatise
1815—Laennec discovers mediate auscultation
1822—Magendie demonstrates Bell's law of the spinal nerve roots
1836—Schwann discovers pepsin
1842—Long operates with ether anesthesia
1843—Holmes points out contagiousness of puerperal fever
1846—Bernard discovers digestive function of pancreas
1847—Helmholtz publishes treatise on conservation of energy
1850—Helmholtz measures velocity of nerve current
1853—Sims publishes treatise on vesicovaginal fistula
1853–56—Crimean War: Florence Nightingale
1858—Virchow's *Cellularpathologic* published
1859—Darwin's *Origin of Species* published
Florence Nightingale publishes *Notes on Nursing*
1861—Pasteur discovers anaerobic bacteria

1867—Lister introduces antiseptic surgery
1875—Meat inspection compulsory in Germany
Public Health Act in England
1876—Imperial Board of Health founded at Berlin
Royal Sanitary Institute founded in London
1882—Koch discovers tubercle bacillus
1888—Pasteur Institute founded
1889—Behring discovers antitoxins
1803—Röntgen discovers X rays
1894—Kitasato and Yersin discover plague bacillus
1899—Reed and Carroll establish transmission of yellow fever by mosquitoes
1900—Blood groups discovered
1903—Electrocardiograph developed by Einthoven
1905—Frozen section method for surgical biopsies developed by Louis B. Wilson
1906—Retrograde pyelography
1913—Supreme Court denies rights inimical to public welfare
1923—Intravenous pyelography
1926—Introduction of continuous intravenous infusion
1928—Fleming isolates *Penicillium notatum*
1932—Intravenous anesthesia comes into use with hexobarbital (Euipan)
1935—Sulfanilomide derivative (Protonsil), active against hemolytic streptococcus, discovered by Domagk
1939—Beginning of surgical correction of cardiac abnormalities with R. E. Gross's ligature of patent doctus arteriosus
1941—Publication of clinical results with penicillin
1942—Curare becomes popular as a muscle relaxant
1943—Hoffman discovers LSD-25

1944—Discovery of streptomycin for tuberculosis

1947—Direct attack on the heart with operation of the mitral and pulmonary valves

1948—Discovery of cortisone

1950—Oxytetracycline produced by A. C. Finlay and a team of ten others

1955—Salk announces development of an effective polio vaccine

1967—Heart transplants in America and Africa

1973—Double-helix model of DNA structure proposed by Watson and Crick

Index